BOOK 6

EMOTIONS AND MIND

The Open University

This publication forms part of an Open University course SD226 *Biological Psychology: Exploring the Brain*. The complete list of texts which make up this course can be found on the back cover. Details of this and other Open University courses can be obtained from the Course Information and Advice Centre, PO Box 724, The Open University, Milton Keynes MK7 6ZS, United Kingdom: tel. +44 (0)1908 653231, e-mail general-enquiries@open.ac.uk

Alternatively, you may visit the Open University website at http://www.open.ac.uk where you can learn more about the wide range of courses and packs offered at all levels by The Open University.

To purchase a selection of Open University course materials visit the webshop at www.ouw.co.uk, or contact Open University Worldwide, Michael Young Building, Walton Hall, Milton Keynes MK7 6AA, United Kingdom for a brochure: tel. +44 (0)1908 858785; fax +44 (0)1908 858787; e-mail ouwenq@open.ac.uk

The Open University
Walton Hall, Milton Keynes
MK7 6AA

First published 2004

Edited, designed and typeset by The Open University.

Printed and bound in the United Kingdom by the Alden Group, Oxford.

ISBN 0 7492 6628 7

1.1

SD226 COURSE TEAM

Course Team Chair

Miranda Dyson

Academic Editor

Heather McLannahan

Course Managers

Alastair Ewing
Tracy Finnegan

Course Team Assistant

Yvonne Royals

Authors

Saroj Datta
Ian Lyon
Bundy Mackintosh
Heather McLannahan
Kerry Murphy
Peter Naish
Daniel Nettle
Ignacio Romero
Frederick Toates
Terry Whatson

Multimedia

Sue Dugher
Spencer Harben
Will Rawes
Brian Richardson

Other Contributors

Duncan Banks
Mike Stewart

Consultant

Jose Julio Rodriguez Arellano

Course Assessor

Philip Winn (University of St Andrews)

Editors

Gerry Bearman
Rebecca Graham
Gillian Riley
Pamela Wardell

Graphic Design

Steve Best
Sarah Hofton
Pam Owen

Picture Researchers

Lydia K. Eaton
Deana Plummer

Indexer

Jane Henley

Cover image: *Anxiety* by Edvard Munch (© Munch Museum/Munch-Ellingsen Group/DACS 2003; Photo: © Munch Museum (Andersen/de Jong))

Contents

CHAPTER

I

MOTIVATION

1.1 Introduction

1.1.1 What is meant by motivation?

In everyday conversation, we all use the term 'motivation'. For example, we speak of someone 'being highly motivated', 'motivated by hunger, fear, lust or greed' or 'lacking any motivation'. It would seem that the opposite of 'being motivated' is being passive in situations where others actively engage, as in a couple of the features of depression: helplessness and withdrawal. So, what *motivates* us into activity? Within biological psychology, motivation refers to a particular set of brain processes underlying the control of behaviour. This set is responsible for the selection of *one particular* behaviour, amongst several possible behaviours, and giving strength, persistence and direction to that behaviour. For example, a hungry person is engaged with thoughts of food and their behaviour is directed to finding food; a frightened person is occupied by thoughts and actions directed to escaping from the fear-evoking situation. The motivation to take drugs is one example that will be considered in this chapter. For example, a smoker might come under the irresistible grip of the motivation to smoke and be said to 'lack the motivation' to quit.

A feature of one motivation can be illustrated by reconsidering the system that controls water intake (Book 1, Section 1.5.3). You may remember from that section that a period of deprivation of water increases both the motivation to seek water and the amount of water ingested when it becomes available.

- ◆ What is the functional significance of increased motivation with deprivation of water?
- ◆ Increasing dehydration is of increasing danger to the physical integrity of the body. By prioritizing the seeking of water, that risk is lowered.

- ◆ Apart from measuring the amount of water drunk, can you think of another way that thirst motivation can be measured?
- ◆ For humans, you could ask them to rate their thirst motivation on a scale of 1 to 10 or ask them the amount that they are prepared to pay to get a bottle of water. Another index, usually applied to rats, is the frequency with which a trained animal will press a lever in a Skinner box (Book 1, Figure 1.23a) for the reward of water. A highly motivated animal will tend to press the lever at a high rate.

There are often several motivations simultaneously present in the brain and thereby forming candidates for taking control of behaviour, for example a person may want to eat and find a source of water. Another example is when an antelope near a waterhole is motivated both by fear of the lack of cover with its associated risk of predation (suggesting withdrawal) and by thirst (suggesting approach). This leads to the notion of competition between motivations for expression in behaviour. In other words, one motivation inhibits the others in a so-called 'winner-takes-all' process – whichever motivation is the most powerful exerts inhibition on the expression of competitors.

Motivation can be applied to the range of activities with which animals, both human and non-human, engage. Some motivations, such as those underlying feeding, drinking and sexual behaviour, are obviously related to the study of biology. However, we need to resist the temptation of trying to divide activities into those that are, or are not, 'biological'. All activities are organized within the CNS. The notion of motivation encourages us to see the common features underlying the organization and control of some very different activities. For example, imagine being torn between visiting friends and staying in to finish a TMA. The concept of motivation draws our attention to competition within the CNS for gaining the control of behaviour and the notion of a dominant motivation that wins (finishing the TMA, of course!).

In biological psychology, things such as food and a sexual partner, towards which behaviour is directed, are sometimes termed 'rewards'. An alternative term and one that emphasizes the behavioural *pull* of such things is **incentive**, and it will be used here. The term incentive is also used to describe locations associated with the primary incentives, such as a location associated with food, e.g. the site in a T-maze (used in Figure 1.11) where food has been found in the past, in that this exerts a draw on the animal at times of hunger.

In the explanation of brain, behaviour and mind, Book 1, Chapters 1 and 4 considered both events within the nervous system and conscious events as reported by introspection. Both these sources of insight are used in understanding motivation. Thus, it has surely not escaped your attention that pleasure is a feature of the expression of human motivation in behaviour, as in sex or eating food while hungry. Pleasure can be linked to homeostasis.

- Can you recall from Book 1, Section 1.2.2 what the term 'homeostasis' means?
- Homeostasis refers to a property of the body that has two aspects. First, the body tends to keep such things as fluid level and temperature within close limits. This is important for survival. Secondly, when such a parameter deviates from its normal level, action is taken to restore normality. This can involve behaviour.

Humans report intense pleasure when homeostatic deficits are reduced – as in drinking when dehydrated. However, discomfort and pain are also features of motivation and motivate a *move away from* the source of the disturbance. Thus, contact with the world that is associated with a move away from homeostasis is aversive, for instance encountering a cold object when body temperature is below normal.

Within psychology, the scientific adjective used to refer to the dimension of pleasure and pain is **hedonic**, as in the expression 'hedonic factor in motivation'. We will be concerned with the pleasure half of this term, for example as used to refer to the human experience of pleasure in eating a tasty food. Thus, a particular neurochemical might exert an effect on hedonics, meaning, for example, that it normally mediates a role in increasing the pleasure associated with eating. The injection of its agonist (a substance that mimics the effect of a particular natural neurochemical) might be associated with increased taste ratings for food. In extrapolating this logic to non-humans, we need caution. Although non-humans cannot give verbal reports of pleasure and pain, it is now commonly assumed that such an experience extends to at least some species. How we might speculatively identify such states in non-humans is described in Section 1.2.4.

As another example of introspection and explanation, consider an addict going out in search of a drug. A particular motivation arising within the brain gives direction to his behaviour. Behaviour is directed to visiting certain parts of town where the drug can be obtained and other competing demands are given a lower priority, i.e. they are suppressed. Behaviour switches to taking the drug after it is obtained. The addict might describe how his conscious mind is occupied with thoughts about drugs, planning how to get them and imagining the 'high'. The term **craving** refers to this occupation of the mind with a desire for something unavailable. For humans, it seems to be at the essence of what we mean by 'motivation'. This exemplifies that two sources of evidence, the objective (e.g. neural events) and the subjective (e.g. the conscious feeling of craving), need to be integrated in forming a picture of human motivation.

This chapter will make extensive use of studies on non-human species, especially rats. This is because the kind of biological measurements and interventions that are needed for gaining insight can only be done on non-humans. In a sense, the rat serves as a 'model system', i.e. we hope that at least some insights gained from rat studies can cautiously be extrapolated to humans.

1.1.2 Types of motivation

There are various types of motivation, some of which are concerned with homeostasis.

- Give examples of links between homeostasis, motivation and behaviour.

- A deficiency of nutrients triggers motivation towards obtaining food and ingested food reduces the deficiency. Loss of body water triggers thirst motivation, fluid ingestion and, subsequently, correction of dehydration. A deviation from the normal body temperature creates a motivation to correct this, for example by seeking either a warm or a cold place, according to the deviation. In each case, homeostatic balance is restored by behaviour and the motivation is eliminated or at least reduced.

Sexual motivation is an example of a conventional motivation that is not normally associated with the maintenance of homeostasis. However, despite a variety of motivations, a notion underlying their study is that they all have something in common. Indeed, this must be the case for the word 'motivation' to have any utility. As a general principle that will be developed later (Sections 1.2.2, 1.2.3 and 1.3.1), both internal events (such as levels of water, nutrients, hormones) and external events (such as food, an attractive partner) play a role in motivation.

This chapter will look at feeding, sexual behaviour and drug taking. It will consider some of the features that are particular to the motivational control of feeding and sexual behaviour. It will also look at some features of motivation that are general across the control of several behaviours. It will then go on to suggest that such general processes can be taken over by addictive drugs.

Motivation and learning are closely linked and so an understanding of motivation requires drawing upon knowledge from learning (Book 5, Chapter 1). Motivation also depends in part upon learning based on experience. For example, cues that in the past accompanied feeding serve to increase feeding motivation. You might feel your appetite increases as you smell something wafting from the kitchen or as you approach a favourite restaurant. An animal can be trained to press a lever in a

Skinner box or run a maze for incentives such as food, water or sexual contact. This procedure is described as utilizing **positive reinforcement** (Book 5, Section 1.2.3), where the frequency of the behaviour increases as a result of its outcome, for example obtaining food. Specifically in the context of instrumental tasks and where learning is revealed, such incentives as food and water are also termed **positive reinforcers**.

The notion of motivation is applied both to behaviour that acts to *gain* something, such as food or water, and where behaviour acts to *avoid* something, for example fear can motivate avoidance such as running to a safe location. Purely for space considerations, this chapter is concerned only with behaviour directed to the gain of something.

1.1.3 Appetitive and consummatory phases of motivation and behaviour

For feeding, drinking and sex, motivation is applied to two phases of behaviour. One phase, the **appetitive phase**, describes actions that lead to the *gain* of something, e.g. food. As examples, consider a human preparing a meal or a rat lever-pressing in a Skinner box or running a maze for food. How does the term 'motivation' help us to understand this behaviour? Behaviour can be characterized by, amongst other things, its strength (i.e. 'intensity'), indexed by how fast the animal runs or how frequently it presses the lever. Food deprivation increases this strength. Deprivation means that a trained animal would be willing (i.e. motivated) to work for food even on a harsh reinforcement schedule (for instance, where only every twentieth lever-press earns a food pellet). The notion of, for example, feeding motivation leads us to investigate the link between:

- events within the body related to energy levels (i.e. physiological events), and
- the organization of behaviour directed towards the gain of food (i.e. behavioural events).

The second phase, the **consummatory phase**, describes what happens after the 'something' sought in the appetitive phase is encountered, as exemplified in the case of food by the act of feeding. One can use 'motivation' here in a similar way to that for the appetitive phase, in terms of the intensity of behaviour. For instance, at the start of a meal there might be a high feeding motivation and a switch to another activity is unlikely. As a substantial amount of food is ingested, there is a reduction in the strength of feeding motivation. This could be indicated by a switch from feeding to something else. Again we are dealing with the process that links physiological events, such as nutrient levels, and behaviour.

Under most conditions, the strength of behaviour exhibited within appetitive and consummatory phases show a close correlation. That is, we tend to want what we like (and consume) and like what we want. Similarly, an animal would normally show a high motivation in terms of both lever-pressing in a Skinner box and the quantity of food eaten. However, the correlation between the strengths of appetitive and consummatory measures is not invariably high. One such example is where an animal works for food that has been devalued by taste-aversion – the Garcia effect (Book 5, Section 1.4.2). In this situation the animal will sometimes work in a Skinner box for such a reward but decline to eat the pellets. Furthermore, there are some different neural mechanisms underlying the appetitive and consummatory phases. A given chemical manipulation will sometimes disrupt one of the phases of behaviour but leave the other intact.

1.1.4 Basic neuroscience of motivation

The 'biological seat' of motivation is assumed to be the neural activity within particular combinations of distinct regions of the brain. For rats, we can alter motivation by manipulations that target specific regions of the brain, as in the case of lesions and chemical interventions. Small amounts of the agonist or antagonist (a substance that blocks the effect of a natural neurochemical) to different neurochemicals can be applied to selected brain regions and their influence observed. Strictly speaking, any behaviour involves the whole brain and all its neurochemicals acting in complex interaction. But are there specific nuclei or neurochemical pathways that have a particular *identifiable* role in motivation?

- What do you think this question means?
- The question directs us to look for particular nuclei or neurochemical pathways that are, for example, especially active when an animal is engaged in lever-pressing for food ('highly motivated'), and inactive when it has ingested a substantial amount ('low motivation').

Damage to these nuclei or neurochemical pathways would be expected to be associated with some loss of motivation.

For humans, PET scans reveal high neural activity in particular brain regions at a time of intense engagement with ('motivation towards') an activity such as playing a video game. This is in addition to, for example, any accompanying increased activity in brain regions known to be concerned with vision.

From various studies on rats and humans, a pathway known to employ the neurochemical dopamine (DA) appears to be a key to understanding motivation. This dopaminergic pathway, termed the **mesolimbic dopaminergic pathway**, projects from a midbrain region, the ventral tegmental area (VTA), to a number of forebrain regions, such as the nucleus accumbens (N.acc.) and the amygdala (see Figure 1.1a and b). As will be described shortly, the activity of the mesolimbic dopaminergic pathway is fundamental to the appetitive aspect of behaviour, i.e. the seeking (and, in humans, 'wanting') aspect of motivation, irrespective of which motivation and behaviour we consider. Thus, in terms of its role, it is described as an **incentive motivation pathway**. If a rat's brain is depleted of DA, the rat shows a loss of appetitive behaviour, such as that directed to feeding.

- Can you recall a role of DA that was discussed earlier in the course?
- DA is involved in the control of motor output. (Parkinson's disease is caused by a loss of dopaminergic neurons that project from the substantia nigra to the striatum (Book 1, Section 1.5.2 and Book 4, Section 1.6.4).)

This dopaminergic pathway (called the 'nigrostriatal pathway') is also shown in Figure 1.1a. This pathway is involved in the organization of motor control. Hence a loss of *all* DA from the brain might not be very interesting from a perspective of motivation, since the rat might cease to eat, for example, simply because it cannot perform the mechanical act of ingestion. However, researchers are able to target particular dopaminergic regions of the brain. They can disrupt the mesolimbic dopaminergic pathway, leaving the nigrostriatal pathway intact. When a DA antagonist is targeted to the mesolimbic dopaminergic pathway, the animal tends to ignore food even though it shows no difficulty in locomotion. This suggests that the pathway has something to do with motivation.

Since the mesolimbic dopaminergic pathway plays a role in various motivated activities it will be discussed in the context of feeding, sex and drug taking. In addition, we will ask how such factors as nutrient deficiency and hormone levels influence specific motivational processes. In the next section we will look at some specific motivations.

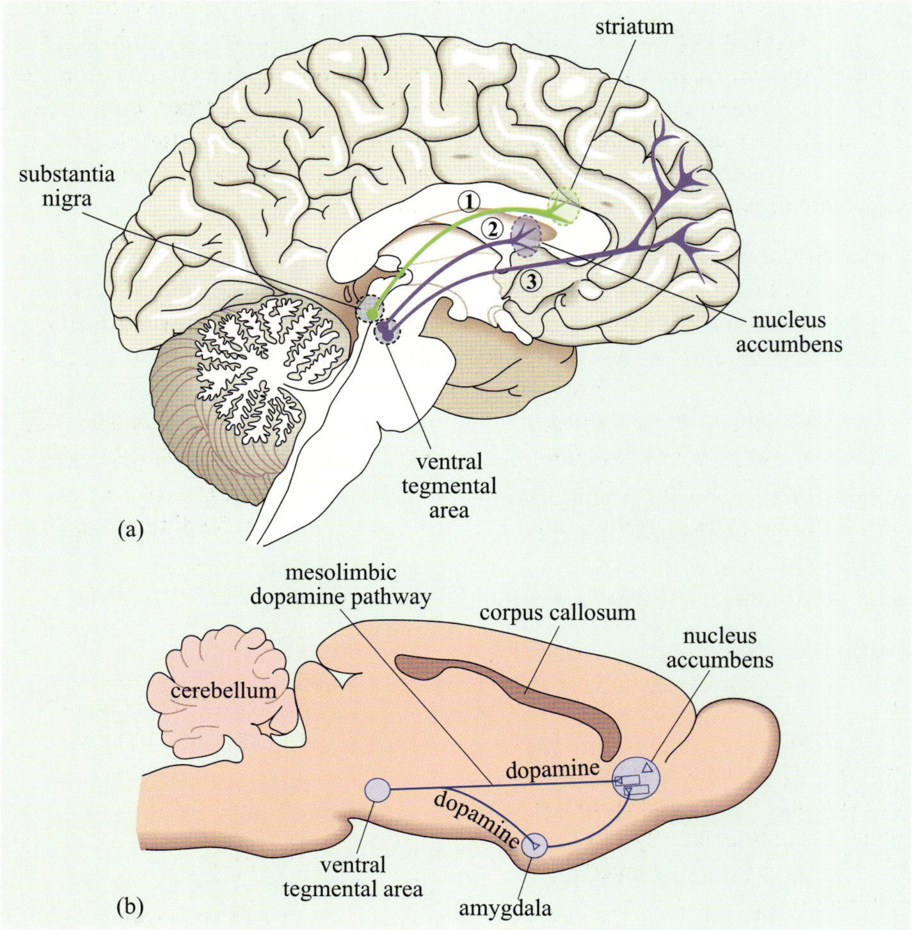

Figure 1.1 The brain's dopaminergic pathways, showing (a) part of the mesolimbic dopaminergic pathway (routes 2 and 3) and nigrostriatal pathway (route 1) in a human and (b) part of the mesolimbic dopaminergic pathway in the rat.

Summary of Section 1.1

The term 'motivation' refers to processes underlying active engagement with the world. This involves selection of a particular candidate motivation in the face of possible competition for control. Motivation applies to appetitive and consummatory phases of behaviour. In some cases, motivation relates closely to homeostasis. The study of motivation involves an integration of objective and subjective ('introspective') evidence. Motivation can be revealed in the context of learning as exemplified by positive reinforcement. One neural pathway that features extensively in accounts of motivation across a number of different examples is the mesolimbic dopaminergic pathway, which projects from the ventral tegmental area to the nucleus accumbens and some other forebrain structures. It constitutes an incentive motivation pathway.

1.2 Feeding motivation

1.2.1 Introduction

This section considers the behaviour of feeding and its underlying motivation. Feeding motivation depends upon both external factors (e.g. the presence of food) and the internal physiology of the animal. There are both excitatory and inhibitory contributions to feeding motivation. The term **appetite** is employed to describe the excitatory contribution to feeding motivation (see Figure 1.2). All other things being equal, as the body is depleted of nutrients there is an increase in appetite. Ingestion of food is associated with an inhibitory effect on motivation termed **satiety**. It acts in the opposite direction to the excitatory effect of appetite.

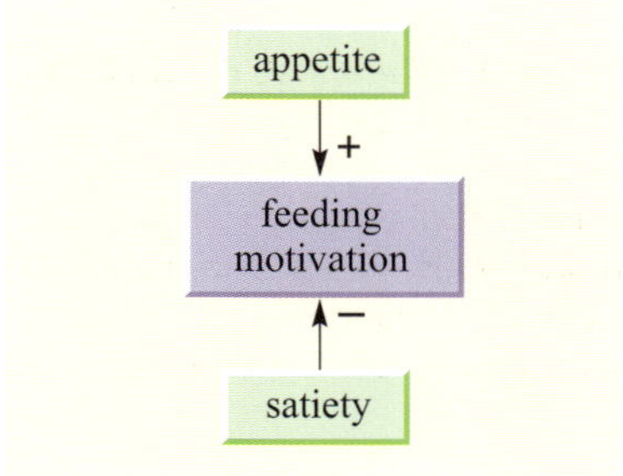

Figure 1.2 Feeding motivation, as determined by the difference between appetite and satiety.

In the following section, we will describe briefly some of the physiological processes of the body that are involved in the ingestion and processing of nutrients. For the purpose of investigating feeding motivation, the term **nutrient state** can be used to describe the level of the various nutrients in the body. So, Section 1.2.2 will first consider some of the events within the body arising from the nutrient state that form the bases of the *internal* contribution to motivation. We will then look at how this relates to the excitation of feeding motivation and how, following ingestion of food, motivation is switched off. In Section 1.2.3 we will look at the role of the incentive stimulus of food itself, i.e. the external contribution, in feeding motivation.

1.2.2 The internal contribution to feeding motivation

Basic biology

Humans (and rats) take distinct meals with pauses between them. Food enters the alimentary tract (the tube that runs from mouth to anus) at the mouth, and then digestion occurs in the stomach and intestine. Absorption of food from the alimentary tract starts shortly after ingestion. Nutrients are conveyed from the wall of the intestine via capillaries and the hepatic portal vein to the liver (Figure 1.3). Following their arrival at the liver, nutrients may be:

- sent immediately in the blood to provide the metabolic needs of tissues throughout the body;
- chemically converted and stored in the liver, e.g. as fat deposits;
- despatched and chemically converted in the periphery of the body, e.g. laid down as fat deposits.

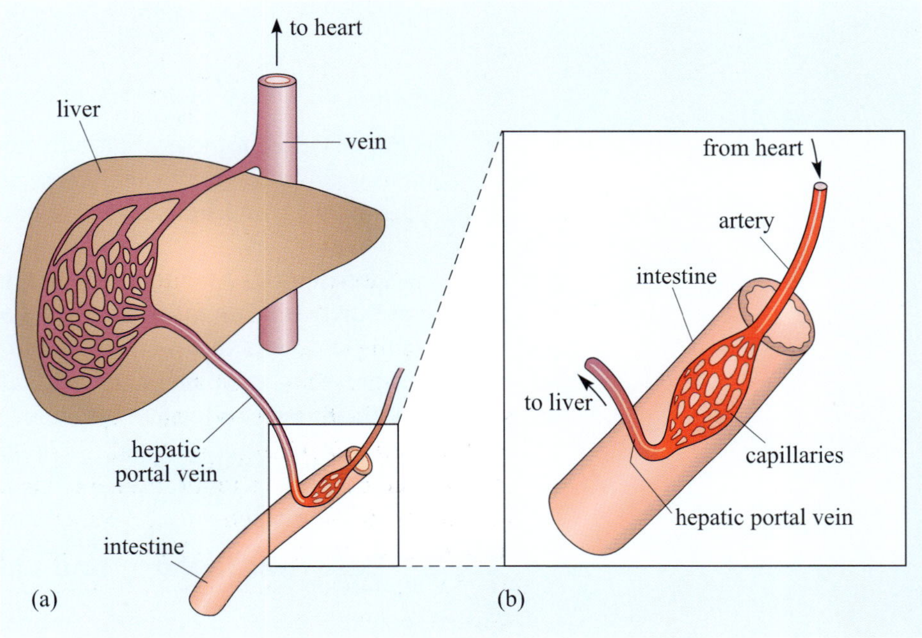

Figure 1.3 (a) Absorption of nutrients from the intestine. (b) Part of (a) shown expanded.

Appetite

In the appetitive phase, the motivation to seek food depends upon signals arising from the nutrient state together with external information arising from food (for instance, the sight and smell, memory of food locations). Additional factors such as the time within the 24 hour period also play a role. In the consummatory phase, information on the nutrient state acts together with direct sensory information on the food itself as perceived by mouth and nose. Subjective reports point to an initial increase in motivation towards tasty food after some of it has been ingested.

Various theories have attached the appetite signal to different features of the nutrient state of the body. Given the variety of chemical transactions and their different locations within the body, which sites and which signals play a role in appetite? At different times in the history of biological psychology, the emphasis has been on a particular factor such as a fall in blood glucose or a fall in the level of stored fats. A contemporary position is that a combination of factors from within the nutrient state is exploited in generating appetite. We investigate this in Section 1.2.4.

Satiety

At first, you might think that if we could identify the internal signal that switches feeding on ('appetite'), the answer to what switches it off would be provided at the same time, i.e. lowering the switch-on signal by ingested food. However, in the case of both feeding and drinking, things must be more complex.

- Why are things more complex than the idea just expressed?
- Food and water are ingested, enter the stomach and then the intestine. Subsequently, they are absorbed across the wall of the intestine and enter the blood. They are then distributed to various tissues, where nutrients are converted chemically. This takes time. Long before all of a meal or drink has been absorbed, most species will have stopped feeding or drinking and will be doing something else.

- How does this observation relate to the motivation signal underlying feeding?
- The combination of factors that switches feeding off ('satiety') appears to be somewhat different from a simple reversal of those factors that switch it on, as is implied by the two distinct arrows in Figure 1.2.

Such considerations lead to the notion that ingestion is switched off by means of a short-term satiety process following ingestion. Satiety arises from a combination of events: in the long term, there is a reversal of the instigating conditions for motivation, but in the short term there are factors such as the act of chewing, stimulation of taste receptors and the bulk of food in the stomach that switch off feeding.

We now turn to a consideration of the role of one of the external factors in motivation: the presence of food.

1.2.3 External factors and their processing

Clearly, potential foods differ in their ability to arouse feeding motivation; some have higher incentive values than others. The contribution of taste to feeding motivation is termed **palatability**. The chemical content of food is detected by receptors located on the tongue and in the nose. Neural signals project from the receptors to brain regions involved in motivation.

Certain associations formed with a particular food can play a role in its subsequent contribution to motivation. For example if the food has been associated with nausea in the past:

- its intake will be lowered (Book 5, Section 1.4.2);
- sometimes (though not always) it is associated with a reduction in appetitive behaviour.

Species such as rats and humans eat a variety of foods. From a functional perspective, there are various nutrients needed to maintain a healthy body and it might not be possible to obtain them all in one food type. Rats and humans satiated on one food can find their appetite revived if there is a change of diet. This shows that a memory of food ingested in the past plays a role in motivation, i.e. information on physically present foods is compared with information on past ingestion. Rats were given a 2 hour test period made up from four 30 minute periods. The various diets A, B, C and D were identical except for the addition of a tiny morsel of characteristic flavouring, such as almond or lemon. You can see from Figure 1.4 that the intake increased on 'variety days' when A, B, C and D were available for 30 minutes each over the 2 hour period, as compared to when the same diet was available for the sequence of four 30 minute periods (e.g. CCCC). Variety, as in many supermarkets, is one cause of obesity. The excitatory effect of variety overrides the inhibitory influences of elevated fat deposits. Viewed in functional terms and in a more natural environment, there is a price that comes with opportunistic foraging for both rat and human. What might sometimes appear attractive could in fact be harmful, e.g. a poisonous berry. This points to the adaptive significance of taste-aversion learning (Book 5, Section 1.4.2).

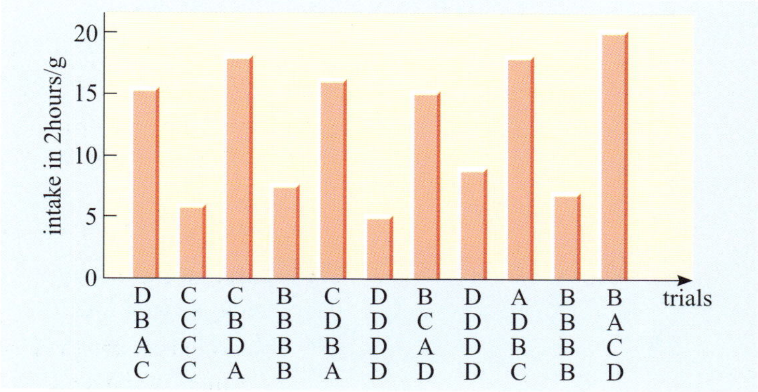

Figure 1.4 The effect of variety in a diet on food intake. Either 'variety' (e.g. DBAC) or 'no variety' (e.g. CCCC) conditions are imposed on alternate days.

In the next section we will look at how the nutrient state of the body and information on food is used by the CNS to provide a motivational signal controlling food seeking and feeding.

1.2.4 The neuroscience of feeding

Introduction

Regions of the brain involved in feeding motivation are informed about the nutrient state of the body as well as about foods in the environment. Some neurochemicals and hormones appear to have a role specifically in feeding motivation, whereas others are exploited in the motivation underlying more than one activity. As an example of specificity, some neurochemicals and hormones are involved in the process of detecting the nutrient state of the body. Other features, of more general use, such as the mesolimbic dopaminergic pathway (Section 1.1.4), are also recruited by the feeding motivation pathway. This section will consider both of these contributions to motivation.

Suppose that the antagonist to a certain natural neurochemical is injected and this produces a decrease in food intake relative to that following a control injection.

- Does this imply that under normal conditions the neurochemical that is antagonized has a specific role in feeding motivation?
- Not necessarily. The natural neurochemical might normally have a general excitatory effect on any motivation and behaviour. Alternatively, the injected substance might make the animal feel ill and thereby depress all active behaviour.

- What kind of control procedure is needed to rule these out as explanations?
- The effect of the injection on other behaviour, such as drinking or sex, could be investigated.

If the antagonist has a specific effect on feeding motivation or behaviour and on nothing else, this would suggest that the neurotransmitter that it antagonizes is specifically involved in feeding motivation.

- What are some of the processes that might be implicated in such a decrease in feeding?
- The neurochemical might be involved in the motivation to seek food, in satiety or in the hedonics of feeding.

Detection of nutrient state

As you know, there are excitatory contributions from nutrient state to appetite. There are also signals that contribute to satiety. What are these signals and how do they influence motivation? There appear to be several internal signals that together produce appetite. One is to do with levels of glucose. Glucose is used by the cells of the body, including neurons, as a source of energy. It appears that when there is a decline in the availability of glucose to certain key neurons in the brain region known as the hypothalamus (Figure 1.5), these neurons change the rate at which they produce action potentials. This change in neural signal contributes to feeding motivation. A fall in the availability of glucose at the liver is another trigger to feeding. Neurons in the liver detect this fall and, by means of neural and hormonal links, convey the information to the hypothalamus. Another input to the hypothalamus is as follows. The substance ghrelin is secreted into blood vessels of the stomach during fasting and is transported in the bloodstream as a hormone. At the arcuate nucleus of the hypothalamus, it attaches to receptors and has an appetite stimulating effect. Another factor that plays a role in feeding motivation derives from a hormone termed **leptin**, which is released by fat cells of the body. A fall in leptin levels is detected at the arcuate nucleus and tends to excite appetite. Thus, the hypothalamus appears to be a site of integration, where different inputs are combined with information arising at the hypothalamus itself, in determining feeding motivation.

Clearly, any motivation signal must be conveyed to those brain regions concerned with the organization of behaviour. For example, by some route, the mesolimbic dopaminergic pathway derives an input from the hypothalamus, hence triggering approach to food-related cues. Similarly, when the animal is ingesting food, those motor pathways involved in organizing the motor act of chewing, etc. derive an input that arises from hypothalamic integration regions.

A hormone, cholecystokinin (CCK), is released from the gut by the presence of food. It is conveyed by the blood to the brain, where it has a satiety-inducing

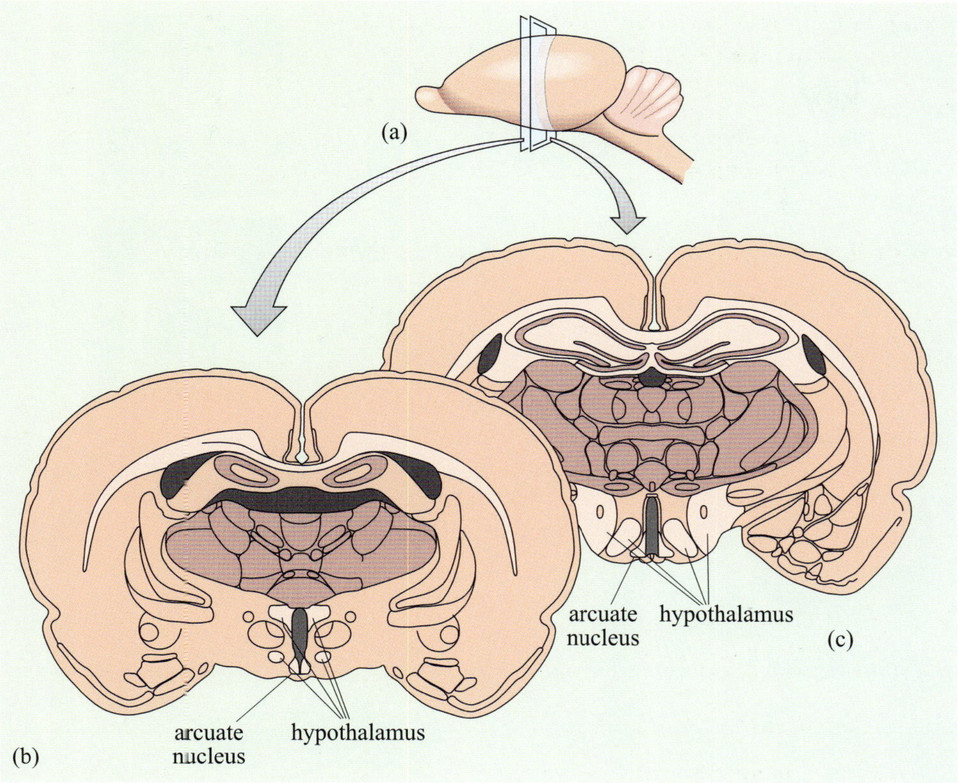

Figure 1.5 (b) and (c) Sections of a rat brain, taken from locations indicated in (a), showing the position of the hypothalamus and its arcuate nucleus.

effect. Given the immense cost to society of obesity, researchers are actively engaged with devising dieting drugs that could mimic satiety without creating nausea.

So much for the specific processes of exciting and inhibiting feeding motivation. We now turn to a consideration of neurochemicals that are more generally exploited across a range of motivations and look at their role in so far as feeding motivation is concerned.

The role of dopamine and opioids

In studies investigating the effect of neurochemicals on feeding motivation, the role of DA and **opioids** has formed one important focus.

The term 'opioid' refers to a class of natural neurochemicals that have close similarities with morphine and heroin. The term **opiate** refers to the 'artificial' (i.e. externally derived) form of the chemical, as in the case of morphine and heroin.

Under natural conditions, opioids have a role in feeding motivation and behaviour. Similarly, as already noted, DA plays a role in a broad range of activities. Manipulations of DA and opioid levels change food intake. We will now look at the role of these neurochemicals in food-intake control.

Disruption of dopaminergic transmission is followed by the loss of intake of food and water. But what exactly is the role of DA in normal food intake? We first consider this role and then that of opioids. Insight into the role of these neurochemicals required the invention of a clever piece of apparatus, described next.

In ingesting food, rats display a range of oral behaviours such as lapping that facilitates the movement of food into the mouth (Figure 1.6a). Human infants also show a range of facial reactions to food (Figure 1.6b). In the **taste-reactivity test**, small amounts of different substances can be placed on the tongues of rats and their ingestive reactions noted (Figure 1.7). This technique eliminates the appetitive phase and reveals the pure consummatory reaction. Its inventors describe it as a technique that reveals the 'hedonics of taste'.

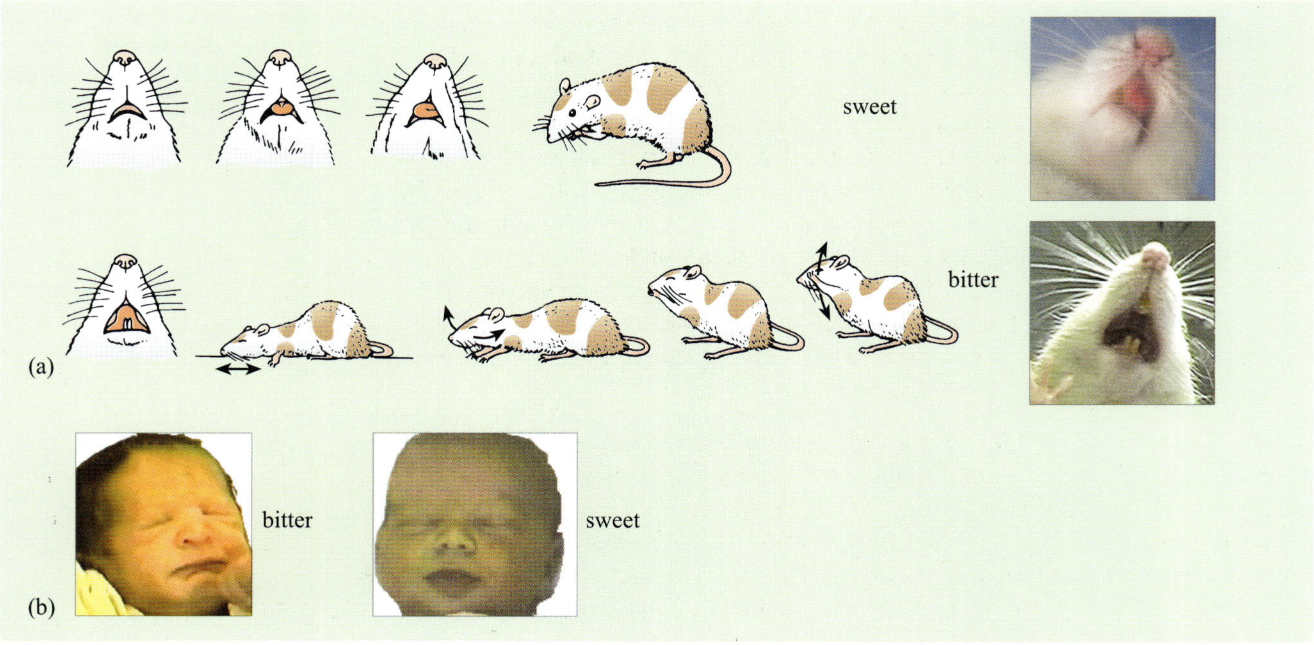

Figure 1.6 Taste reactions of (a) rats and (b) human infants to attractive and aversive substances. Arrows indicate sweep of rat's head movement.

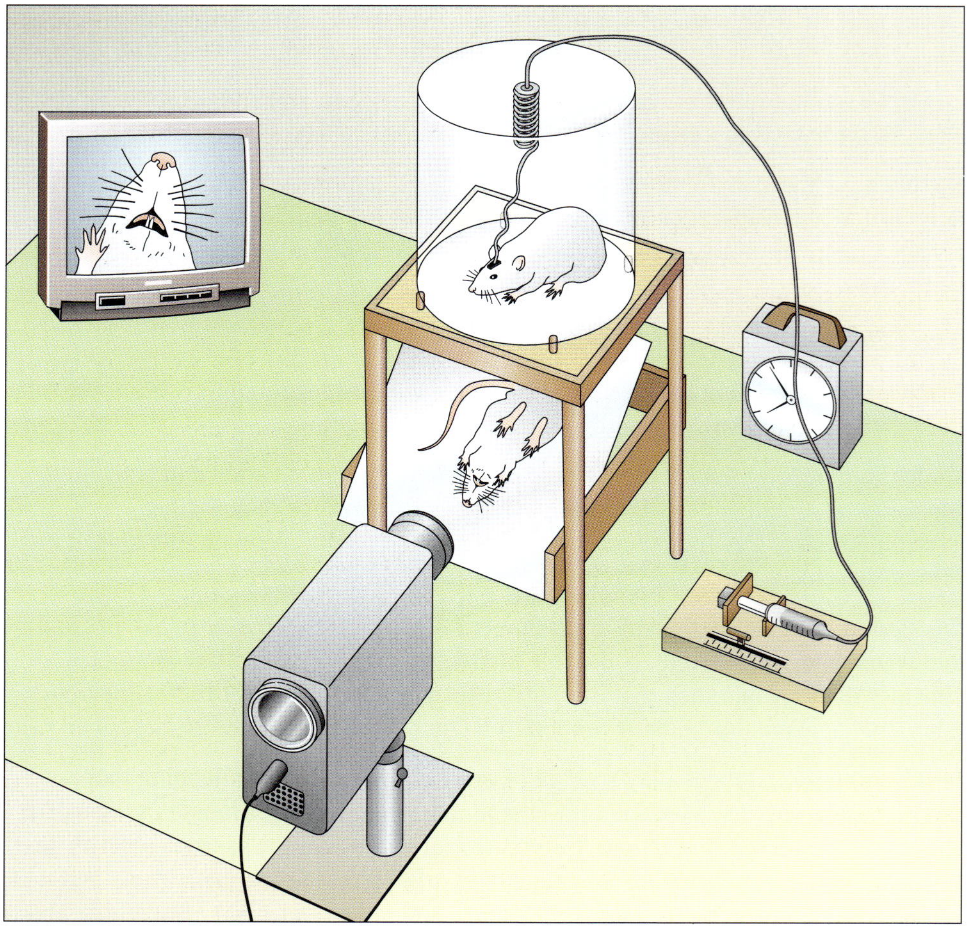

Figure 1.7 Taste-reactivity test showing syringe, tube and micropipette as well as the apparatus for recording and displaying the rat's reactions. The mirror shows the underside of the rat.

Substances that humans describe as 'hedonically positive' trigger a sequence of 'acceptance' reactions. This sequence maximizes ingestion in both rats and newborn infants. Substances that are described as 'unpleasant' trigger a quite different sequence of reactions (termed 'rejection' reactions), such as those to avoid or escape contact. Neutral substances elicit both acceptance and rejection reactions. The reactions change in a way that makes sense from the perspective of homeostasis. For example, a strong solution of sodium chloride (salt) normally triggers an aversive reaction. However, if the rat is in salt deficiency, the same solution triggers a positive (acceptance) reaction. Suppose that intake of a saccharine solution, which normally triggers a positive reaction, is followed by nausea. Subsequently, the same solution triggers an aversive reaction, as if it tastes bad. This indicates taste-aversion learning.

So, by what process does the injection of antagonists to DA disrupt food intake? One influential theory, the 'anhedonia hypothesis' (i.e. loss of hedonia), is that the hedonic value of food depends upon the integrity of the mesolimbic dopaminergic pathway (Figure 1.1a and b). With the loss of this pathway, food loses its hedonic impact. It is difficult to test this hypothesis in humans. Parkinson's disease involves a depletion of the nigrostriatal pathway and so does not give clear insight here. However, the invention of the taste-reactivity test provided the means to test the role of DA in rats.

- ◈ If the anhedonia hypothesis is true and rats with disruption of the mesolimbic dopaminergic pathway are tested with normally acceptable food, what would be the prediction?
- ◆ The pattern of reactions would be less positive, in other words a move from predominant acceptance to more rejection.

In fact, researchers found that the pattern was unchanged following such disruption. Hence the anhedonia hypothesis was not supported. In other words, the *liking* of food appeared to be unaltered with the loss of the mesolimbic dopaminergic pathway. There was also little support for the idea that the mechanics of ingestion were disrupted, since the same motor reactions were shown as before the disruption of the mesolimbic dopaminergic pathway. Since dopamine-deficient rats slow up and then stop responding on instrumental tasks rewarded with food, it was concluded that appetitive behaviour was disrupted, i.e. DA plays a role in the attraction of an animal towards food (the 'incentive value' of food). Loss of DA results in a loss of motivation directed to food. The suggestion was made that distant cues associated with food (e.g. smell, visual cues) become attractive as a result of activation of the mesolimbic dopaminergic pathway. A change in diet is associated with the activation of this pathway.

Of course, if DA is not involved in the hedonic process then some other neurochemical is involved. A strong candidate is an opioid substance since the injection of opiates at the time of ingestion shifts taste reactivity in a positive direction, i.e. in the acceptance direction. Opioids are also involved in pain; for example injection of the opiate morphine reduces pain. Several pieces of evidence point to the release of opioids being triggered by the ingestion of palatable food, especially sweet-tasting food, and contributing to the hedonics of taste. In one study, the reaction of human infants to blood collection by syringe was measured. The amount of crying was less if they were given a bottle with a solution containing sugar as compared to plain water just prior to the injection.

- What possibility does this result suggest?
- It suggests opioid substances were released by the sugar taste and this lowered pain and negative emotional reactivity.

- What kind of evidence would support this possibility?
- If the effect of the opioid substance was blocked by an opioid antagonist, which indeed it was in the study.

In rats and humans, the injection of opioid agonists increases food intake, whereas antagonists decrease it.

- What caution should be exercised when trying to interpret the effects of antagonists?
- The antagonist might reduce feeding by means of a non-specific effect such as nausea.

In fact, only a few human participants do report nausea following injection of an opioid antagonist. The opioid antagonist naltrexone reduces the preference for sweet tastes in humans and decreases the reported liking of foods. Figure 1.8 shows the effect of naltrexone on hunger ratings during the course of eating a portion of pasta with cheese sauce or a more highly rated tomato sauce.

- Interpret what you see in Figure 1.8.
- Naltrexone does not affect hunger ratings at the start of either of the meals. Naltrexone decreases intake relative to baseline and placebo conditions for both foods. If it is assumed that feeding is terminated when satiety counters appetite, this point occurs earlier as a result of the naltrexone injection.

This result is compatible with studies on rats, indicating that opioids play a role in calculating the hedonic effect on motivation of ingested food. Opioids appear to have no effect on motivation prior to ingestion.

- How might this be tested in rats?
- The effect of opioid antagonists on the frequency of lever-pressing under extinction conditions could be examined as this is a measure of motivation unaffected by food intake. In addition, the size of a meal eaten could be measured. This is a possible index of an hedonic effect.

The result of such an experiment is that opioid antagonists have little or no effect on lever-pressing in extinction but do reduce the size of a meal.

The nucleus accumbens is a site where injected opioid agonists have a particular role in increasing food intake. Such results led researchers to conclude that opioids are involved in the rewarding or hedonic aspects of food intake. That is, their effect is to increase the hedonic assessment of food and thereby increase intake.

Learning also plays an important role in determining intake. Cues associated with feeding come to acquire the capacity to trigger dopaminergic activation and ingestion.

- This is an example of what form of learning?
- Classical ('Pavlovian') conditioning (Book 5, Section 1.2).

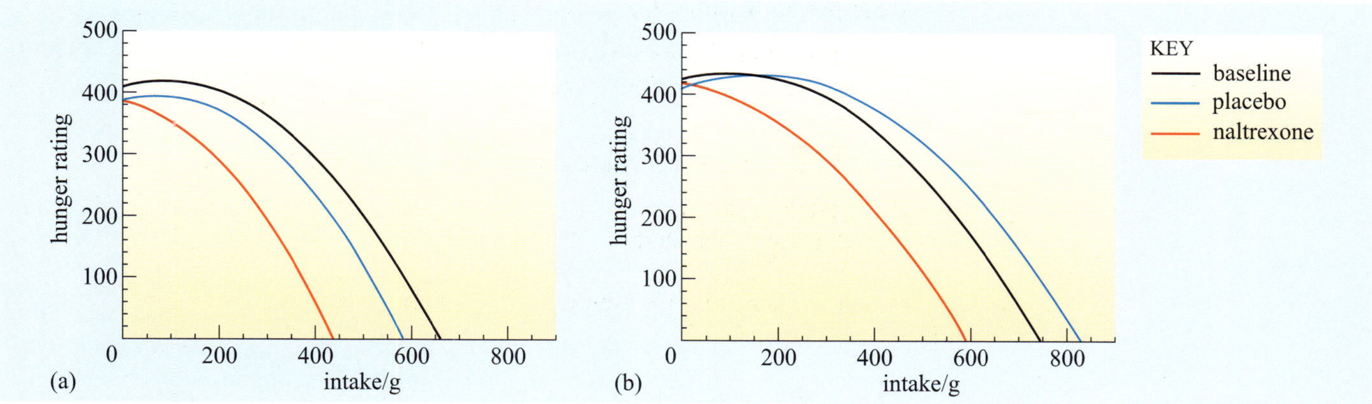

Figure 1.8 Hunger ratings as a function of amount ingested for (a) pasta with cheese sauce and (b) pasta with a more highly rated tomato sauce.

Summary of Section 1.2

Feeding motivation arises from a combination of internal factors (e.g. levels of blood glucose, leptin) and external factors (food, cues paired with food). Appetite describes the positive contribution to feeding motivation. Satiety refers to the process that switches off feeding motivation and arises in part from short-term consequences of ingesting food. Increases in motivation can arise from changing the available diet. DA plays a role in the appetitive phase of feeding motivation. Opioids have a role in computing the hedonic value of food that is being ingested.

1.3 Sexual motivation

1.3.1 Introduction

Sexual motivation and behaviour are triggered by a combination of an external stimulus, an incentive (i.e. a potential mate), and internal factors. The internal factors are made up of, for example, hormones that affect neurons in regions of the brain such as particular nuclei of the hypothalamus (but different nuclei from those involved in feeding motivation). For example, testosterone is a hormone secreted by the male testes and the adrenal gland in both sexes and then transported in the blood. At the brain it affects the activity of target neurons that are sensitive to its presence. These neural processes play a specific role in sexual motivation and behaviour. There are also appetitive and consummatory phases of sexual behaviour. This section will look at a few features of these phases.

1.3.2 Sexual desire

Human sexual motivation ('desire') can be 'measured' by subjective reports (i.e. how aroused someone feels) and indices such as the rate of blood flow within the genital region (termed 'engorgement'). Most of the research on humans as well as on rats has been carried out on male sexuality and so that is reflected here.

Human sexual desire and behaviour are so strongly determined by cultural and social factors that it is difficult to isolate the role of specific biological factors. However, the hormone testosterone has a primary role in facilitating sexual desire in both women and men (provided other conditions are also met, such as the presence of a partner or thoughts of one). Thus, the term 'male sex hormone', widely used in the popular literature to describe testosterone, is somewhat misleading.

Testosterone also has a developmental effect (Book 3, Section 3.3.3) in the early formation of regions of the CNS that will have a role in later sexual motivation and behaviour.

In adolescent boys, testosterone levels correlate with their reported frequency of sexual thoughts and levels of sexual activity.

- What caution needs to be sounded before assuming that higher levels of testosterone play a role in triggering sexual thoughts and behaviour?
- The difficulty of establishing cause and effect. The levels of testosterone could be increased by sexual thoughts and activity. Indeed, one might expect a reciprocal interdependence between (a) hormone levels and (b) thoughts and behaviour, i.e. each affects the other (Book 1, Section 1.3.3).

In one study, it was found that exposure of males to a film of specifically erotic content increases their levels of testosterone.

- What sort of control condition is needed in such a study?
- Looking at neutral images is one control condition, but this would not control for emotional arousal of a non-sexual kind. Humorous or violent video clips would provide some control for general emotional arousal.

Research points strongly to the existence of a causal link between the presence of the hormone and sexually related cognition and behaviour. For example, in men that have been surgically castrated, cessation of the supply of testosterone is followed by a reduction in the frequency of sexual thoughts, and intensity of sexual desire and activity. Replacement of testosterone using an exogenous (meaning 'from the outside') source is followed by a reversal of these changes.

In women, surgical removal of the adrenal glands (for instance, as a treatment for cancer) is often followed by a sharp drop in sexual desire, which can be restored by administering exogenous testosterone. It is sometimes argued that oestrogens have relatively little direct effect on sexual desire in either men or women. However, testing this is notoriously difficult since so many factors could play a role. For example, any natural effect of cyclic levels of oestrogens on women's sexual motivation might be masked by the use of contraceptive pills or by cognitive factors ('insight') relating to the probability of pregnancy. Research on lesbian couples points to some variation in desire over the menstrual cycle, with a peak at the time of maximum fertility. There can also be an indirect effect of oestrogens on sexual motivation. At the time of the menopause, loss of oestrogens can be associated with a loss of genital engorgement and lubrication. Pain during intercourse can result, with a corresponding loss of desire.

PET imaging has revealed that in males sexually aroused by presenting them with erotic images there is activation in regions of the brain traditionally associated with emotional processing (Chapter 2). These regions are sometimes given the name 'limbic system' and include the amygdala (Book 1, Section 3.4.4). Testosterone is taken up by neurons at various parts of the CNS, including the amygdala, where it has a stimulating effect on sexual motivation.

As regards neurochemicals, DA plays a role in both the appetitive and consummatory phases of sexual behaviour of various species. As you saw earlier, DA has a role in feeding motivation and so this, together with the evidence in the present section, points to its general effects in the range of motivations. DA agonists have a stimulating effect on sexual motivation, particularly if applied locally to the nucleus accumbens, again pointing to the central importance of this structure in motivation. Appetitive sexual behaviour is disrupted by DA antagonists. Testosterone and DA interact: testosterone enhances the effect of DA in brain regions underlying sexual motivation. In male rats, loss of sexual interest as a result of castration can be reversed by injections of a DA agonist. DA antagonists used for treating mental illness depress the male sexual desire.

1.3.3 The appetitive and consummatory distinction

By means of lesions, researchers have investigated the neural systems that underlie the control of sexual behaviour in rats. This section will consider the role of two regions of the brain: the amygdala and a nucleus of the hypothalamus – namely the medial preoptic area (mPOA) (Figure 1.9).

- ◈ Which dopaminergic pathway projects, amongst other structures, to the amygdala?
- ◆ The mesolimbic dopaminergic pathway.

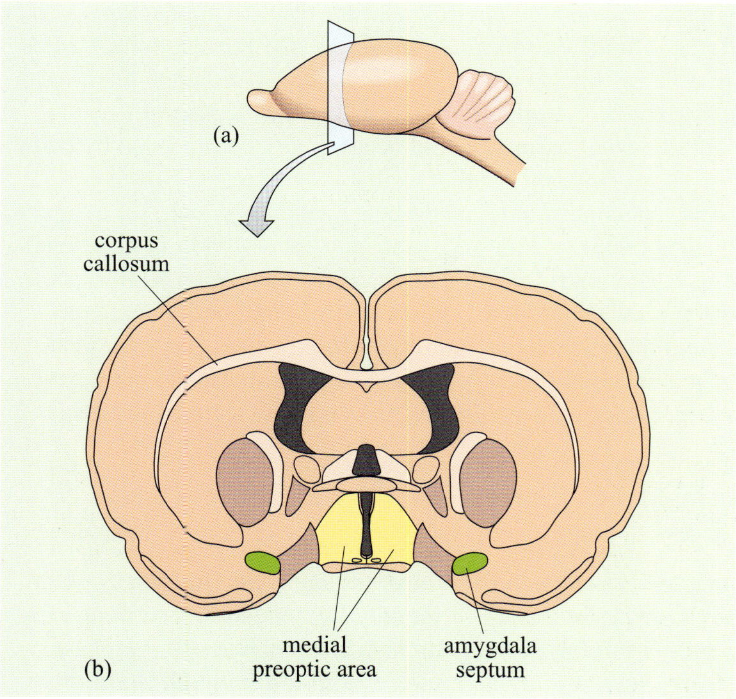

Figure 1.9 (b) Section through a rat brain at the location indicated in (a) showing the position of the medial preoptic area of the hypothalamus and the amygdala.

In one study, a male rat was first trained on an operant task (lever-pressing) to earn the reward of having a female rat introduced into the cage with him and a mating opportunity. A flash of light stimulus accompanied the delivery of reward, i.e. the introduction of a female. Following training, the rats in the experimental group were subjected to a lesion to part of the amygdala. The rats in the control group did not suffer any damage to the brain. Subsequently, the reward of the female was omitted in both groups and only the light was presented following a lever-press. Lever-pressing was considered to be a measure of pure appetitive behaviour. In the control animals, the frequency of lever-pressing remained high immediately after only the light was presented. Compared to the controls, animals that had lesions of the amygdala showed an immediate sharp drop in the frequency of lever-pressing. However, these rats did not show any disruption of their consummatory behaviour – they mated like normal rats when actually in the presence of a female.

This study, along with other evidence, led the researchers to conclude that the amygdala is implicated in associating motivational value to otherwise neutral stimuli, e.g. a tone or light paired with the primary incentive.

◆ What is this process an example of?

◆ Classical ('Pavlovian') conditioning (Book 5, Section 1.2).

◆ Book 1, Section 1.4.2 mentioned the ethological approach to the study of behaviour. What are its central features?

◆ A range of different species is studied. This is done either by looking at the animals living in their natural habitat or by trying to recreate natural features of the environment in the laboratory. Speculation is triggered, thereby raising questions concerning the function of behaviour.

So, what could be the functional significance of the conditioning just described? After all, it must be unusual in a natural environment for the arrival of sexual partners to be heralded by a flash of light! Furthermore, the cues used for recognition of an animal of the opposite sex (e.g. odour) would not normally depend upon learning. A number of possibilities might be considered. It is possible that, in the rat's natural environment, the arrival of sexual partners could occasionally be preceded by certain idiosyncratic sounds or visual changes peculiar to that environment. However, perhaps more likely, classical conditioning could be a means by which, for example, the power of an established odour or auditory stimulus is increased in motivational strength as a result of its earlier pairing with mating. This could be an additional means of triggering the animal's motivation and directing behaviour towards the primary sexual incentive. Finally, such classical conditioning of sexual behaviour might simply reflect a general conditioning process that is more usually employed in, say, associating food (e.g. grain) with particular cues (e.g. the sight of a sack).

There are neural connections by which motivational information computed at the amygdala is conveyed to the nucleus accumbens. This information is further processed and gains access to motor output and thereby the control of behaviour.

Studies have shown that lesions of the mPOA have the opposite effect to those of the amygdala. That is, they disrupt the mating of the rat (e.g. its capacity to mount the female and perform penile insertion) but they do not disrupt the appetitive phase, as indexed by lever-pressing. Such a study is termed a **double-dissociation**. In other words lesion x disrupts behaviour X but not behaviour Y, whereas lesion y disrupts behaviour Y but not behaviour X. A double-dissociation is powerful evidence in linking aspects of behaviour with particular brain regions.

◆ Why is this?

◆ It indicates a selective and specific effect. By contrast, suppose that we know only that a lesion (x) disrupts behaviour X but not Y. It could be that X is very vulnerable to any disruption whereas Y is invulnerable. It could be that intervention (x) has a range of effects and X is just the first to show disruption. The double-dissociation shows that this cannot be so and reveals specificity.

1.3.4 The Coolidge effect

The expression **Coolidge effect** (named after the US president) refers to the fact that, in a number of species, a sexually satiated animal shows a revival of mating if there is a change of partner. The origin of the term is a part of the folklore of psychology and is as follows. One day, President and first lady Coolidge were visiting a farm. For the purpose of the tour, the presidential party was split into two groups, the president in one group and the first lady in the other. On noticing a cockerel that was very sexually active, Mrs. Coolidge asked whether he was so energetic all day. The answer she got was that he mated dozens of times each day. Mrs. Coolidge replied, 'Please tell that to the President.' Later, the President reached this point on the tour and the cockerel was pointed out to him. The president asked, 'Same hen every time?' and was told, 'Oh no, Mr. President, a different one each time.' President Coolidge then made the remark for which he was destined to be immortalized in biological psychology, 'Tell that to Mrs. Coolidge!'

- From a functional perspective, in a species such as the rat or human, what sense does the Coolidge effect make?
- Being attracted to mating with multiple partners might be a means whereby an animal's genes are spread more widely.

What kind of mechanism underlies this? Clearly it involves a memory of past mating and a comparison of incoming sensory information with this. Researchers have investigated whether DA release in the nucleus accumbens is triggered by the presentation of a novel female rat to a sexually 'satiated' male. They employed the technique of *in vivo* microdialysis (Book 3, Section 2.4.1). An increase in DA release and renewed appetitive and copulatory behaviour were triggered by the novel female, suggesting a DA basis of this behaviour.

Although the Coolidge effect has long been a part of the folklore of behavioural science, on close examination, experiments designed to detect its presence confront quite horrendous problems of control. You might like to consider what these are.

So much for natural, biologically adaptive examples of motivation and behaviour. In the next section, we turn to an example that would seem to be decidedly non-adaptive.

Summary of Section 1.3

Sexual motivation arises from a combination of external factors, an incentive (e.g. a potential mate and cues that have been paired with one) and internal factors. The hormone testosterone plays a crucial role in the appetitive phase of sexual behaviour. Studies on rats point to the amygdala as being closely involved in the appetitive phase of sexual motivation whereas the medial preoptic area is involved in the consummatory phase. A change of partner can re-arouse sexual motivation, a phenomenon termed the Coolidge effect. Dopaminergic pathways are involved in the appetitive phase of sexual motivation.

1.4 Addiction and psychoactive drugs

1.4.1 Introduction

The term **addiction** is commonly employed to refer to the compulsive use of **psychoactive drugs** (drugs that exert a psychological effect). Excessive amounts of time and effort are devoted to the pursuit of a drug by some people, even when this appears to be to the overall detriment of the person. However, 'addiction' can also be employed to describe other activities that consume large amounts of time or which do not appear to make rational sense. Thus, there are such expressions as, 'It's not love – it's more an addiction', 'I wish he were not so addicted to the Internet' and 'I am a chocoholic and I feel like a drug addict needing her fix.' Just what it is about an activity that means we feel justified in using the expression 'addiction' is not entirely clear. Usually, there is the implication of an element of irrationality in the activity in terms of its negative effects on health and well-being, its intensity or the length of time spent on it, or some combination of these. Thus, one criterion is that the addiction creates a problem that is in need of resolution.

From a scientific perspective, can we define 'addiction'? If we generate a definition, does this restrict it to the use of drugs or can we extend it to other behaviour? As is often the case in biological psychology, theorists agonize over how to define a particular term. This section will show where biological psychology can give insights into the processes that underlie addiction.

Clearly, addiction is an example of motivation taking an abnormal direction and so the study of the general principles of motivation is needed to understand it. Reciprocally, understanding addiction is of relevance to understanding the general principles of motivation, since it exemplifies how behaviour can be captured for extended periods of time by one particular motivation.

- In seeking an animal model of addiction, certain drugs are described as 'positive reinforcers'. What might be meant by this term in the context of drug taking?

- An animal will learn to perform an operant task for the reward of intravenous drug or injection through microelectrodes implanted in the brain. That is, presentation of the drug makes the immediately preceding behaviour of lever-pressing more likely to occur.

This section will take a broad look at some activities that can become addictive, with an eye to describing some general principles of the biology underlying them. But first, it is necessary to consider some of the issues that surround a definition of addiction.

1.4.2 The criteria for addiction

Introduction

The classic example of a criterion used to define addiction is the behaviour shown towards drugs such as heroin. However, there are certain other drugs that are also taken for their psychoactive effects but which are not addictive – ecstasy and LSD are two examples, and marijuana is not usually found to be addictive. Conversely, some non-drug-related activities can take on serious addictive properties, as exemplified by gambling. So what could drugs that are addictive, as opposed to those that are not addictive, have in common? Could this property also apply to such things as gambling?

Conventional lay understanding and traditional theorizing within psychology often suggest that, at first, substances are taken for reasons such as peer pressure, curiosity and pleasure. Subsequently, for some individuals, a downward spiral of addiction ensues with occasional use giving way to compulsive and destructive use. In reality, only a fraction of the people exposed to potentially addictive substances develop an addiction. A number of people use hard drugs regularly without evidence of craving, disruption or withdrawal symptoms. However, some 15% of people will have developed an addiction to cocaine within a period of up to 10 years after their first use.

The expression 'addiction' is something like that of 'moral goodness': we all use it and we feel that we know what it means, but producing a watertight definition is exceedingly difficult. This section looks at some possible criteria that can be used to define addiction. If all the criteria are met, we would feel confident in using the term. We will also look at the benefits and limitations of employing these criteria. In this context, we consider what biological psychology might be able to contribute.

Excessiveness and disruption

A possible definition of addiction is in terms of the excessiveness of the activity (e.g. in terms of money spent) and the disruption to the life of the addict and others. This can be applied across a spectrum of activities, both drug related and drug unrelated. It gives a pointer to an essential characteristic of our quarry. A problem arises in defining when 'excessive is excessive'. There would seem to be no objective index. However, the notion of the activity being excessive according to *what the person desires* would seem to be a crucial feature of addiction. If the person wants to give up the activity and tries to resist but without success, this would seem to be a useful indicator of the presence of an addiction. It offers the possibility of a theoretical integration across diverse addictions such as to drugs, gambling and sex.

Craving

Someone might be said to be addicted to something if in its absence they report an excessive craving for it. This has the benefit of breadth; it can cover addictions to drugs and such non-drug addictions as shopping, gambling or sex. People commonly report cravings for particular foods, as exemplified by women during pregnancy. It would be difficult to imagine an addiction that was not associated with excessive craving. In this sense, the phenomenon provides a useful clue. Reciprocally, certain other activities are neither described as addictive nor associated with craving. For example, in the absence of LSD, the regular user does not experience a constant and uncomfortable awareness of the missing drug.

◆ Can you think of a possible animal model of craving?

◆ Since craving is defined in terms of reports of the contents of conscious awareness, one cannot find an entirely convincing animal model. If, however, we consider seeking a drug in its absence to be one feature of craving, then there is a possibility. This is the operant behaviour of a rat in a task that was earlier rewarded with a drug but where extinction conditions have now been applied and the rat is still lever-pressing.

On the one hand, human craving is unseen and we only have the word of the so-called addict as to the existence of their craving. Can we base a definition on something unobservable? Of course, we also have the problem of defining 'excessive'. This might be considered a matter of opinion and taste. On the other hand, if the addict reports being seriously disturbed by their craving, this suggests that, for the purpose of treatment, it can usefully be employed as an index of addiction and subsequent recovery. Also, PET scans now enable us to image the brains of addicts at times of craving with useful insight. In one study, craving was deliberately triggered by presenting images of cocaine-related acts such as preparing the drug. The control condition consisted of presenting images that were not drug related. Compared to the control condition, on seeing drug-related images, addicts revealed excitation in brain regions concerned with motivational and emotional processing, such as the amygdala. So, we shall include the phenomenon of craving in our explanation of addiction but try to understand it in terms of its biological roots.

Tolerance

A feature of addictive drugs is that with repeated use the amount of drug needed to gain a given effect can increase. This is known as **tolerance** and it reflects changes in the CNS processes underlying drug taking. A possible index of addiction is when a person needs more and more of a drug to gain the same effect.

Withdrawal symptoms

A fourth approach to a definition of addiction is based on objective evidence of **withdrawal symptoms**. Withdrawal symptoms are uncomfortable and disrupt behaviour. If they are triggered when the person suddenly ceases to engage in their behaviour, then they might be used as a pointer to addiction. Another term in common use and meaning much the same as 'addicted' is to say that withdrawal symptoms are indicative of a person's 'dependence' upon a drug. For such drugs as heroin, withdrawal symptoms consist of, for example, sweating, nausea, cramps and convulsions. According to the traditional account, the pleasure caused by heroin is at first intense but then declines and the frequency and strength of aversive withdrawal symptoms increase. There is no set of identical symptoms following cessation of any addictive drug. Each has peculiar features but all are described as unpleasant and undesired. Some of these can be objectively measured and so the term addiction has meaning in describing a set of symptoms. It does not depend upon the subjective reports of the addict. Based on physiological evidence, alcohol and nicotine can also be associated with symptoms of withdrawal.

According to a definition in terms of withdrawal symptoms, once strongly addicted, it is the attempt to eliminate these symptoms that explains most of the craving and compulsive behaviour. Alas, neither is this definition without its problems. Only a small percentage of addicts that have returned to hard drugs give withdrawal symptoms as their reason for relapse. Somewhat surprisingly, times of the most potent cravings do not correlate strongly with times of withdrawal. Detoxification programmes fail to cure a significant percentage of those attending. Similarly, in the case of nicotine, there is no strong relationship between withdrawal symptoms and relapse of smoking. Nicotine replacement, which reduces the withdrawal symptoms following cessation of smoking, is of only very limited help in giving up.

The criterion of withdrawal in defining addiction would appear to be applicable only to certain drugs and thereby preclude, say, Internet addiction or compulsive shopping. However, even a drug such as cocaine might not qualify as being addictive in that there is relatively little in terms of observable withdrawal symptoms – and yet by the criterion of craving and disruption to life, it can be highly addictive.

Withdrawal symptoms are also inadequate to explain how something analogous to human addiction is exhibited by rats. Suppose that a group of rats are trained in a

Skinner box to earn intravenous drug until they could be described as 'dependent', i.e. cessation of availability of the drug is associated with withdrawal symptoms. They are then 'rehabilitated' by being taken off the drug until all signs of withdrawal are lost. What is likely to make them resume lever-pressing? Researchers compared two situations. First, the effect of triggering withdrawal symptoms by injecting the opioid antagonist naltrexone was investigated. Secondly, there was the procedure termed **priming**. This consisted of a small amount of the drug that had previously been earned by lever-pressing being delivered 'free' by the experimenter (when the rat is not in a withdrawal state). The latter procedure was far more effective than the former in triggering resumption of lever-pressing, suggesting that a positive effect of the presence of the drug (or related cues) dominates drug-motivated behaviour.

From a perspective of biological psychology, all addictions necessarily involve changes in the CNS. However, only some (e.g. heroin) are also associated with identifiable changes outside the CNS such as disturbances in the intestine. In this area, a goal is trying to find common features that could apply across the spectrum of addictions. Therefore, of necessity, our focus will be on the CNS. Since drugs can be studied in non-humans, they form an important focus of study.

1.4.3 The neurobiological bases of addiction

Under the heading of addiction, we include a number of chemicals that are taken by humans for their mood-altering properties. These are cocaine, alcohol, amphetamines, nicotine and opiates such as morphine and heroin. Some general principles apply to addictive drugs.

1. Addictive drugs exert their influence by means of direct effects on the brain.
2. By their occupation of receptors on neurons, addictive drugs change the activity patterns of parts of the brain. This is the basis of the psychological changes that follow drug taking. All drugs act on multiple sites within the CNS and have multiple effects. The attraction of drugs would seem to involve a combination of different effects. However, there is some overlap in the effects of addictive drugs and this can be exploited in obtaining an understanding of addiction involving common features shared by these substances.
3. As part of their effects on the nervous system, drugs act on and usurp neural systems that are normally involved in conventional motivational activities such as feeding and sex.
4. Those drugs that are described as addictive for humans are also those that serve as positive reinforcers for rats.

A principal focus in addiction is the mesolimbic dopaminergic pathway (Figure 1.1), sometimes called the 'incentive pathway'. As described earlier, this incentive system underlies the appetitive phase of motivation, which is normally directed to such things as sex and food. All addictive substances (for instance heroin, alcohol, nicotine, caffeine) have the capacity to increase activity in this system. Conversely, a psychoactive substance that is non-addictive, such as LSD, does not target this system. It is relatively easy to track activity in the incentive system in non-humans exposed to addictive drugs. There is nothing that provides a rat model of Internet or gambling addiction! However, evidence obtained from imaging in humans suggests that there is activation in this system when humans engage in an activity such as playing video games.

Certain changes in the nervous system triggered by drugs outlast their immediate psychological mood-altering effects, i.e. there are long-term changes in the properties of neural systems underlying motivation. If drug taking becomes compulsive, then this change is significant, such that drug seeking can come to dominate behaviour. One question we need to address is: what is the nature of this fundamental change in the CNS? But before we answer this question, we need to consider the effects on the nervous system and the behavioural effects of some of the better-known types of drugs.

1.4.4 Some drug types

Introduction

This section considers some types of drug that can be associated with addiction and describes some of their common properties, including the sites within the CNS where they exert their effects. These properties form the basis of a biological theory of addiction. The drugs described range from the strictly illegal to those that form a perfectly legal and normal feature of many of our lives.

Opiates

The drug class termed 'opiates' includes heroin and morphine. They are very similar to substances produced naturally by the body (endogenous opioids or endorphins). Opiates occupy receptors that would, under certain conditions, normally be occupied by their endogenous equivalents. Opiate drugs lock onto opioid receptors that are located at various sites in the nervous system such as the nucleus accumbens (Figure 1.1). They exert various effects such as the relief of pain (discussed briefly in Book 1, Section 1.1.7) and mediating the delights of palatable food (Section 1.2.4). In terms of biological function, pain relief would normally be mediated by endogenous opioids and would help the animal to remain inactive, exemplified by recovering from illness. As witnessed by addicts as well as occasional users and those receiving medication, opiates have the effect not only of easing pain but also of lifting negative emotion and enhancing positive emotion.

There are opioid receptors on the dopaminergic neurons in the nucleus accumbens. On occupying these receptors, opiates increase the release of DA.

- ◆ How might a psychoactive effect of opiates be tested in an animal model?
- ◆ The animal's willingness to press a lever in a Skinner box to earn an injection of drug could be tested.

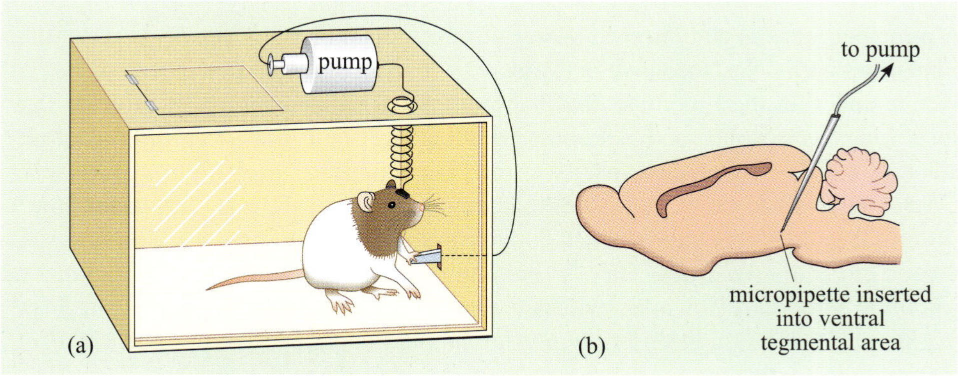

Figure 1.10 Self-infusion through a micropipette: (a) apparatus; (b) cross-section through rat brain indicating micropipette with tip at the VTA.

In one procedure, the apparatus consists of a pump containing opiates, a tube running to the animal and a **micropipette** that is attached to the animal's skull (Figure 1.10a). Rats learn to press a lever to obtain even very small amounts of opiates through such a micropipette when the tip is located in the VTA. Damage to the DA neurons or a microinjection of a DA antagonist to the nucleus accumbens impairs such self-administration of drugs by rats.

Another technique is to see whether an animal shows a preference for the side of a maze associated with experimenter-administered infusion of opiates. Under the control of the experimenter, a single pairing of such an injection and a distinctive environment can cause the rat to choose this environment in the future. This is called a **conditioned place preference** (Figure 1.11).

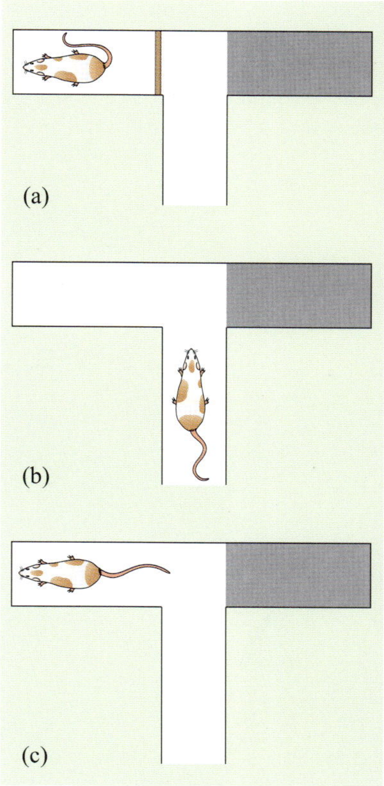

Figure 1.11 Conditioned place preference test. (a) The rat is injected with drug whilst it is in the white arm of a T-maze; (b) the rat is then released from the start and (c) its preference measured by recording the time spent in each arm.

The importance of classical conditioning in the motivation underlying drug seeking is illustrated in the following experiment on rats. Rats are first trained to earn intravenous heroin by lever-pressing in a Skinner box. This response is then extinguished.

- How would the response be extinguished?
- Omitting the drug reward but keeping the rat in the Skinner box until it stops lever-pressing.

The rats are then presented with cues that in the past were paired with the drug. These cues cause excitation of neurons in the nucleus accumbens and reinstate lever-pressing. This might model a phenomenon well-known to drug takers: contexts that in the past were paired with the drug represent a danger for relapse.

Cocaine

Cocaine is associated with subjective reports of pleasure and a 'high'. What is the biological basis of this experience? Cocaine blocks reuptake of DA into the neurons from which it was released (Book 4, Box 1.2). It does this by its attachment to the DA transporter (see Figure 1.12b). Hence, DA is not removed from the synapse as fast as it would normally be. This increases the levels of DA in the synapse and the occupation of DA receptors on the postsynaptic membrane. PET (Book 3, Section 2.4.1) allows the dynamics of cocaine activity to be measured in the human brain. Researchers have compared levels of the drug in the brain following administration of cocaine or methylphenidate. The latter drug is similar in some respects to cocaine in that it blocks DA reuptake. However, it is much less addictive. Labelled cocaine or labelled methylphenidate was injected intravenously into groups of human participants. Figure 1.13 shows PET images at the level of the basal ganglia following the injection of drug. The level of drug in the brain rises following injection and then falls as it is broken down, as can be seen in Figure 1.14. A comparison of the quantity of drug in the brain and the subjective report of 'high' is shown.

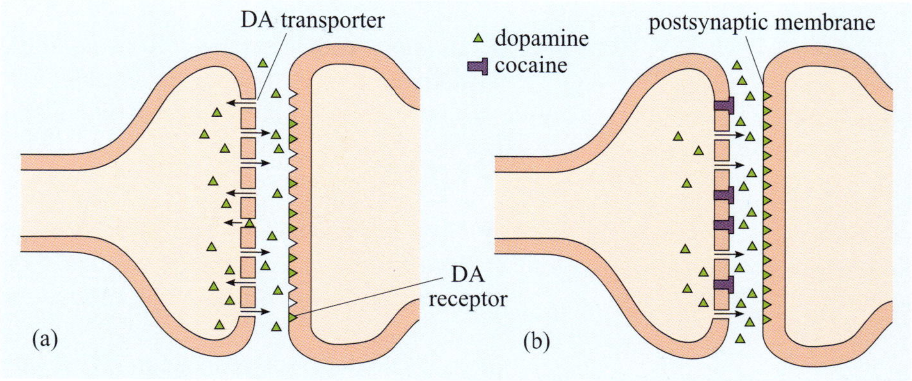

Figure 1.12 Reuptake of dopamine (a) prior to injection of cocaine and (b) following injection of cocaine. Note the blockage of reuptake, increased levels of DA in the synapse and occupying receptors in the postsynaptic membrane.

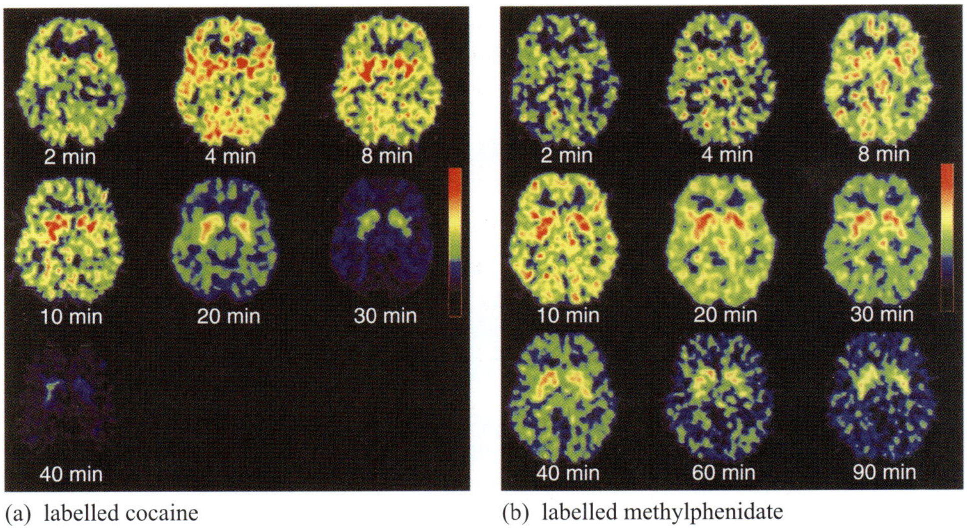

Figure 1.13 PET scans of the human brain at the level of basal ganglia of (a) labelled cocaine and (b) labelled methylphenidate. Red = high values; blue = low values.

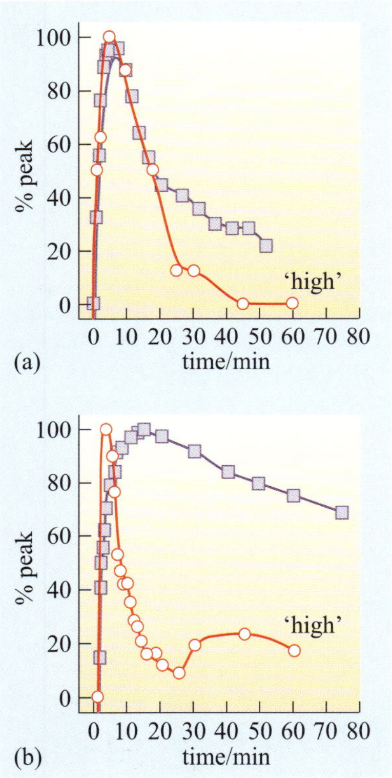

Figure 1.14 Presence in the brain at the level of the basal ganglia and associated subjective 'high' following injection of (a) labelled cocaine and (b) labelled methylphenidate. Red circles = subjective feeling ('high'); mauve squares = drug quantity.

- Interpret what you see in the graphs in Figure 1.14.
- For cocaine, the 'high' follows rather closely the uptake and clearance of the drug in the brain. For methylphenidate, the 'high' declines rapidly in spite of there being significant continued occupation of receptors in the brain.

- Given that cocaine is more addictive than methylphenidate, what is the possible implication of Figure 1.14 for the addictive potential of a drug?
- It suggests that addictive potential is associated with a rapid rise and fall in the level of drug in the brain.

It is interesting to note that typical cocaine binges consist of taking the drug repeatedly at 20–30 minute intervals, hence it would seem repeating the dynamics shown in Figure 1.14a.

Alcohol

Of the various effects of alcohol, those on dopaminergic and opioidergic neural pathways have formed an important focus. Both dopaminergic and opioidergic neural pathways show increased activity as a result of the chemical action of alcohol.

Commonly, people suffering from addiction to alcohol report that their attempts to abstain are thwarted either by negative moods (e.g. stress) or by exposure to cues that have been paired in the past with alcohol (drink-related objects and events).

- Does this represent a clear distinction in the types of trigger?
- Not necessarily. In some cases, drink-related cues will be experienced at the same time as a negative mood. Also, in some cases, a negative mood might serve as a cue that in the past has been associated with alcohol consumption.

In a 'rat model', it is possible to investigate the factors that trigger a relapse to alcohol seeking. In one experiment, the roles of two factors were studied. One of these was the stress experienced by the animal after it had stopped responding for alcohol. The other factor was the presentation of a cue that in the past had been paired with alcohol consumption. First, rats were trained in a Skinner box to earn alcohol. Reward was accompanied by the brief presentation of a distinctive light. They were then placed on extinction conditions until they stopped responding. Finally, under the control of the experimenter, they were exposed to one of three conditions:

1 Stress in the form of a mild shock to the foot.

2 An alcohol-related cue (the distinctive light).

3 Both conditions 1 and 2 combined, with the cue shortly following the mild shock to the foot.

The results are shown in Figure 1.15.

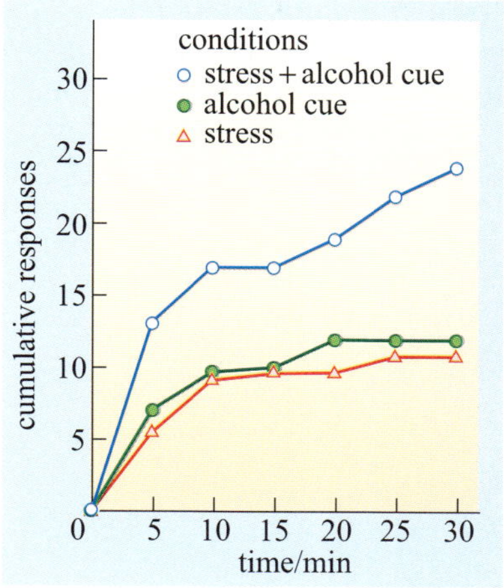

Figure 1.15 Lever-presses triggered (cumulative responses) in the session following completion of extinction (cessation of responding) and in response to the introduction of various stimuli.

- Interpret what you see in Figure 1.15.
- ◆ Each stimulus has the effect of triggering lever-pressing. There is an additive effect when the two stimuli are applied together.

The effect of the conditional stimulus (alcohol-related cue), but not that of stress, was eliminated by administering the opiate antagonist naloxone.

- What is the implication of this result?
- ◆ That an alcohol-related stimulus exerts its effect through the release of endogenous opioid substances. The stressor exerts its effect through some other route.

This result suggests the following. There are chemical effects triggered by alcohol following its ingestion. An otherwise neutral cue paired with alcohol is able, even on its own, to come to trigger some of these same effects. The evidence here points to the role of opioids in this effect.

Caffeine

Caffeine is thought to be the world's most widely taken psychoactive drug. Caffeine has a similar structure to a natural neurotransmitter, adenosine. Activation of adenosine receptors tends to suppress the release of neurotransmitter from those neurons that possess such receptors. Because of its structural similarity to adenosine, caffeine binds to receptors for adenosine in the CNS. However, in so doing, it prevents the normal action that would follow occupation of these receptors. Dopaminergic neurons (Figure 1.16) and glutamatergic neurons also possess adenosine receptors. One effect of caffeine is to increase the levels of both DA and glutamate in the nucleus accumbens. Apart from in coffee, caffeine is found in soft drinks, of which Americans consume enormous quantities. Manufacturers claim that caffeine is added as a flavouring agent whereas controlled trials show that few people can even detect its presence at the permitted concentrations.

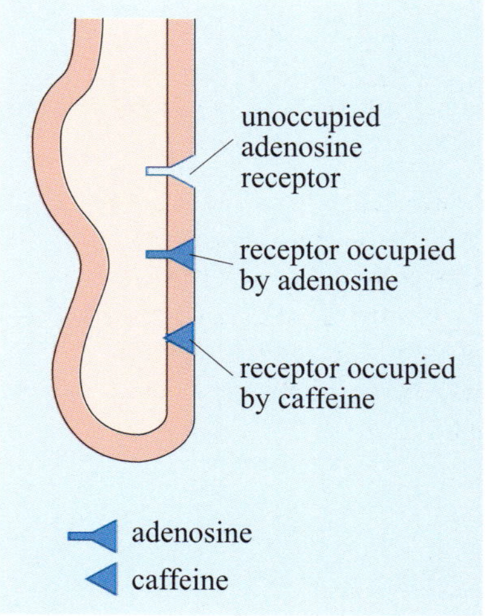

Figure 1.16 Occupation of the adenosine receptor by caffeine.

- Does this mean that manufacturers are wasting their time in adding this ingredient, in that caffeine has no effect on the attraction of such drinks?
- ◆ No. The lure has to be explained somehow. By its effects following ingestion, one might expect caffeine to increase the attraction of products that contain it.

Indeed, an overnight withdrawal symptom from soft drinks is evident in those who consume large amounts.

Nicotine

The primary component of cigarette smoke that maintains the behaviour of smoking is nicotine. Via the lungs and bloodstream, inhaled nicotine reaches the brain within a few seconds. This rapid increase in nicotine in the brain is believed to be associated with the higher addictive potential of smoking as opposed to taking nicotine in gum or via a transdermal patch. Particularly important in this regard is an increase in DA activity in the nucleus accumbens and amygdala that is triggered by nicotine.

The sharp rise in nicotine levels rapidly following inhalation sets the scene for classical conditioning (Book 5, Section 1.2.1) to occur. In other words, cues associated with smoking, such as taste, tactile and visual stimuli, and stimulation of the respiratory system, form an association with the effects of nicotine on the CNS. Such cues are linked to the motor acts of puffing and inhaling. The frequent and repetitive nature of smoking permits a large number of such pairings to occur. This is believed to be a crucial factor in why it is so difficult to stop smoking. The ability of nicotine to satisfy craving in smokers is much less if the upper respiratory tract is anaesthetized. When a smoker is in a context of smoking, such as a bar full of smokers, craving is commonly triggered.

Animal models illuminate the psychoactive effects of nicotine. Thus, rats prefer a T-maze arm associated with nicotine injection. In another model, various species have been trained to self-administer nicotine. The acquisition of self-administration is disrupted by chemical lesions that disturb DA transmission in the nucleus accumbens.

Nicotine withdrawal symptoms in humans, consisting of, amongst other things, irritability and anxiety, are familiar both to those trying to give up smoking and to their families, friends and colleagues. Something analogous appears to exist in rats for which nicotine administration has been terminated. They show an avoidance of the side of a T-maze associated with withdrawal. They also show an elevation in the magnitude of the 'acoustic startle reflex', which is an index of anxiety. Rats resume nicotine seeking after being returned to an environment previously associated with the gain of nicotine. Finally, in rats, stress is a potent trigger to the resumption of nicotine seeking, offering a possible model of the human experience that stress can trigger a resumption of smoking.

Nicotine attaches itself to a type of cholinergic receptor widely distributed in the CNS, termed the 'nicotinic receptor' (nAChR) (Book 4, Section 2.7.1). The addictive potential of nicotine might therefore be due to action at various sites within the CNS. For example, people give one reason for smoking as being 'increased attention'. However, there is reason to believe that the primary site of action that is responsible for its addictive potential is at nAChRs on the DA neurons projecting from the VTA to the nucleus accumbens (Figure 1.1). Infusion of a nicotinic antagonist into the VTA decreases nicotine-seeking behaviour. Blocking of DA transmission by selective DA antagonists applied to the nucleus accumbens greatly reduces lever-pressing for intravenous nicotine and blocks a conditioned place preference for a location associated with nicotine. Nicotine also triggers opioidergic neurotransmission and presumably thereby causes a feeling of well-being. Some (albeit very limited) success at treating smoking has been obtained using the opioid antagonist naloxone.

Smokers commonly report a link between smoking and coffee drinking. There is a positive correlation between cigarette smoking and caffeine intake. It is said that coffee has the effect of triggering smoking since smokers smoke more cigarettes during times of coffee availability.

- ◆ How could this operate?
- ◆ It could be because of the chemical content of coffee. It could be the context in which coffee is taken, for instance after a meal and at a time of social contact. Both might act together.

- ◆ Is it logical to draw a sharp distinction between the chemical content of coffee and context? If not, why not?
- ◆ It is not logical. The effects of coffee post-ingestion will probably set the scene for classical conditioning to occur such that some of the post-ingestive effects on the motivational processes underlying smoking come to be triggered by the taste and sight of coffee.

In rats, the frequency of responding on an instrumental task rewarded with intravenous nicotine was increased by putting caffeine in the drinking water after 14 days (Figure 1.17b), as compared to 'neat' water throughout the same period (Figure 1.17a). The operant task reinforced with the reward of nicotine was the rat poking its nose in a hole. There were two such holes, one termed 'active' that activated the infusion and the other termed 'passive', with no associated consequence. The number of nose pokes and thereby rewards earned were noted.

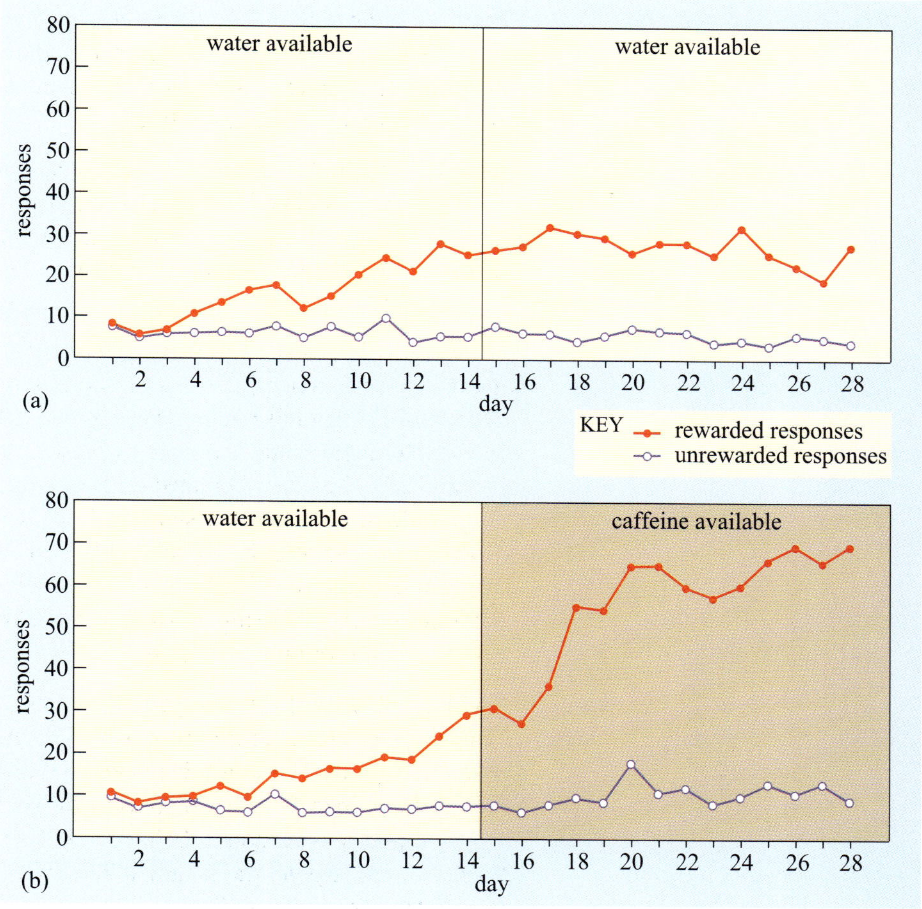

Figure 1.17 Responses rewarded with nicotine (red line) and unrewarded responses (mauve line): (a) with water available throughout; (b) with the water switched to a solution of caffeine after 14 days.

- ◆ Why was a passive hole employed? How did the result comparing responses at the 'active' and 'passive' holes enable researchers to argue specifically that caffeine increases the *reinforcement* value of nicotine?
- ◆ The passive hole served as a control for general increased activity. Note the result shows that increased activity was specifically directed at the 'active' hole.

Figure 1.18 shows a set of results from humans. Smokers received injections of either nicotine or placebo at times of either caffeine availability or caffeine deprivation. As can be seen from the figure, the rating of the effect of the drug injection is higher for the large doses of nicotine when there is a background of caffeine intake.

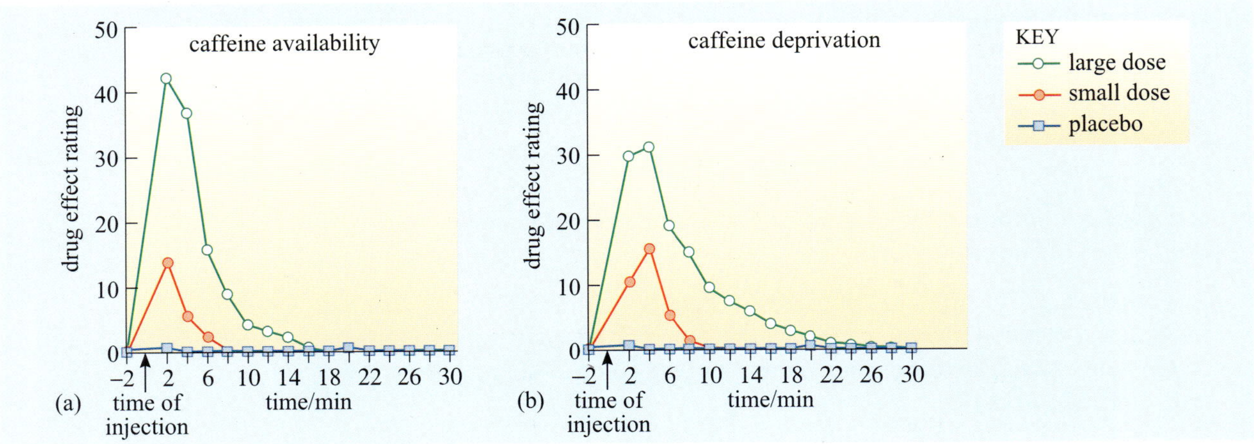

Figure 1.18 Impact of nicotine at times of (a) caffeine availability (b) caffeine deprivation.

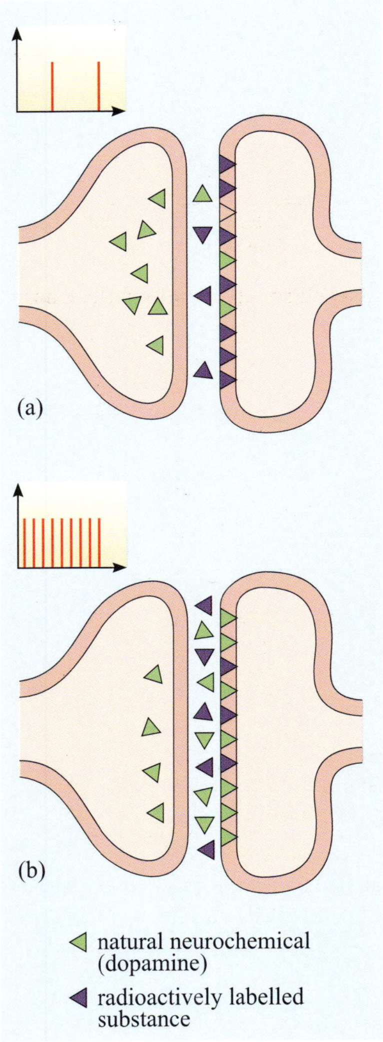

Figure 1.19 Occupation of receptors by injected substance when the natural transmitter dopamine is relatively (a) inactive and (b) active. The small graphs show action potential frequencies within the DA neuron.

- Why might the effect of caffeine on smoking be still greater than this in everyday life?

- Under the experimental conditions providing the results in Figure 1.18, there was no associated action of smoking. In real life, sensory cues such as the taste and smell of a cigarette would be expected to increase the effect.

Common features of addictive substances

In considering some addictive substances, at least two common features emerge:

- various drugs increase the activation of dopaminergic and opioidergic neurotransmission;
- the effects of drugs readily show classical conditioning.

A consideration of these common features means that we can make sense of why, for example, coffee drinking can increase the risk of smoking. Also, it is not difficult to see why smoking cigarettes could trigger, for example, opiate seeking in someone trying to give up opiates. The nicotine would trigger pathways shared with the opiate-seeking processes.

So much for chemicals taken into the body, but what about other forms of addiction? A possible common feature between chemicals that can take on addictive properties and a non-chemically based activity is considered next.

1.4.5 A non-chemical activity

Ideally, a comprehensive account should be able to address activities that do not involve drugs but which can nevertheless become addictive, such as gambling and playing video games. Using a PET scan, researchers looked at the dopaminergic activity of the brain during the playing of a video game. Figure 1.19 illustrates how this was done. Suppose that a labelled substance that occupies DA receptors is injected into a human. This substance competes for binding sites with DA released from neurons. If there is an increase in release of DA, there will be a lower level of occupation of DA receptors by the radioactively labelled substance. Eight participants were asked to learn to 'navigate a tank' in order to earn a reward of money. Figure 1.20 shows the results for the striatum (a region containing the nucleus accumbens) and the cerebellum.

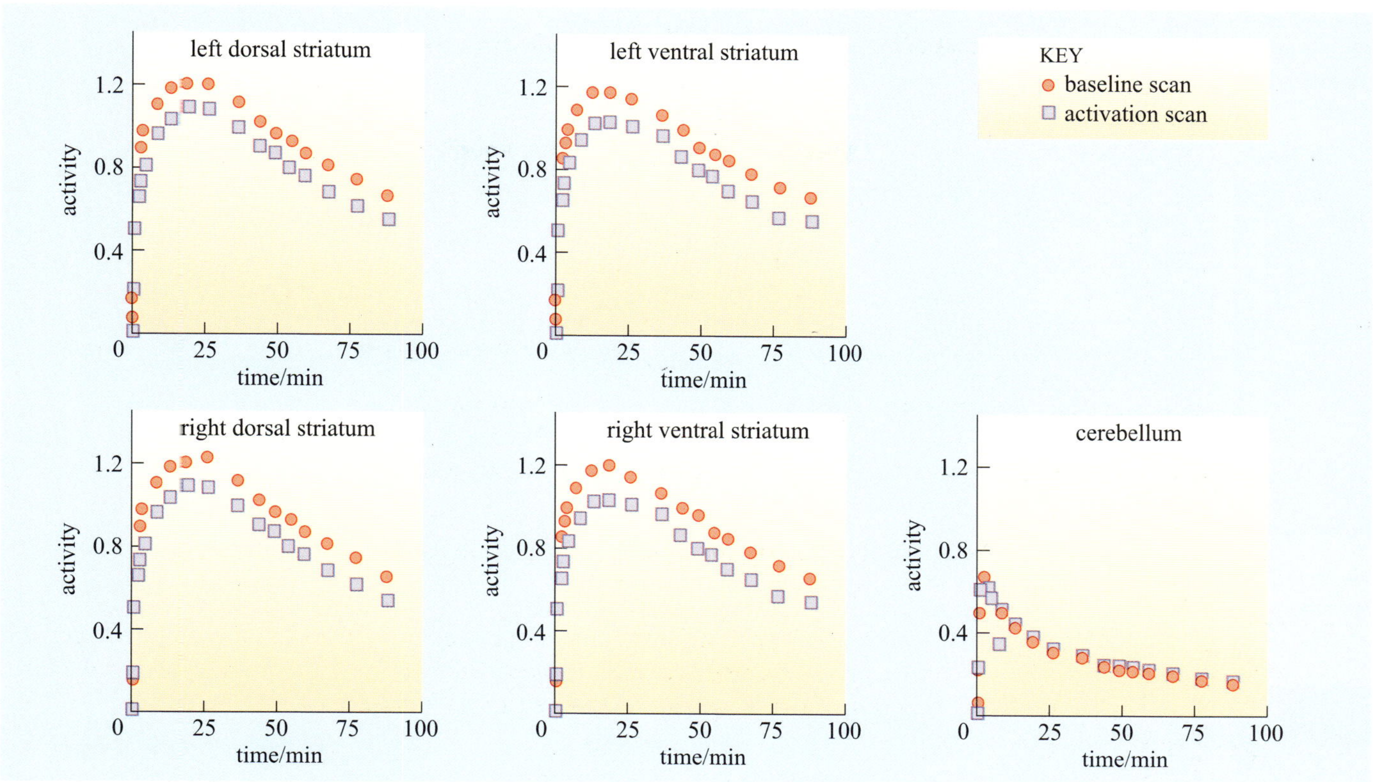

Figure 1.20 Activity curves for radioactively labelled substance in four regions of the striatum, and cerebellum taken whilst participants were playing a video game or in the control condition.

- What do the graphs show in Figure 1.20?
- In the striatum there is a lower occupation of receptors during the performance of a video game ('activation scan') as compared to the background level ('baseline scan').

- What does this suggest concerning DA activation?
- There is an increase in DA release in the striatum during performance of the game.

- Why was activity in the cerebellum also investigated?
- As a control condition to see whether the effect is general or confined to certain brain regions.

- What does the result for the cerebellum show?
- There is a rapid appearance of the radioactively labelled substance in the cerebellum and then a decline, indicative of breakdown. There was no difference between the playing and non-playing conditions.

The researchers compared the performance level of the eight participants with their percentage change in 'binding' (occupation of receptors) between task and baseline conditions (Figure 1.21). A negative correlation between these was found. That is to say, comparing participants, the better they were at the task, the lower was their binding. This points to a possible causal link between level of DA release and successful negotiation of a task.

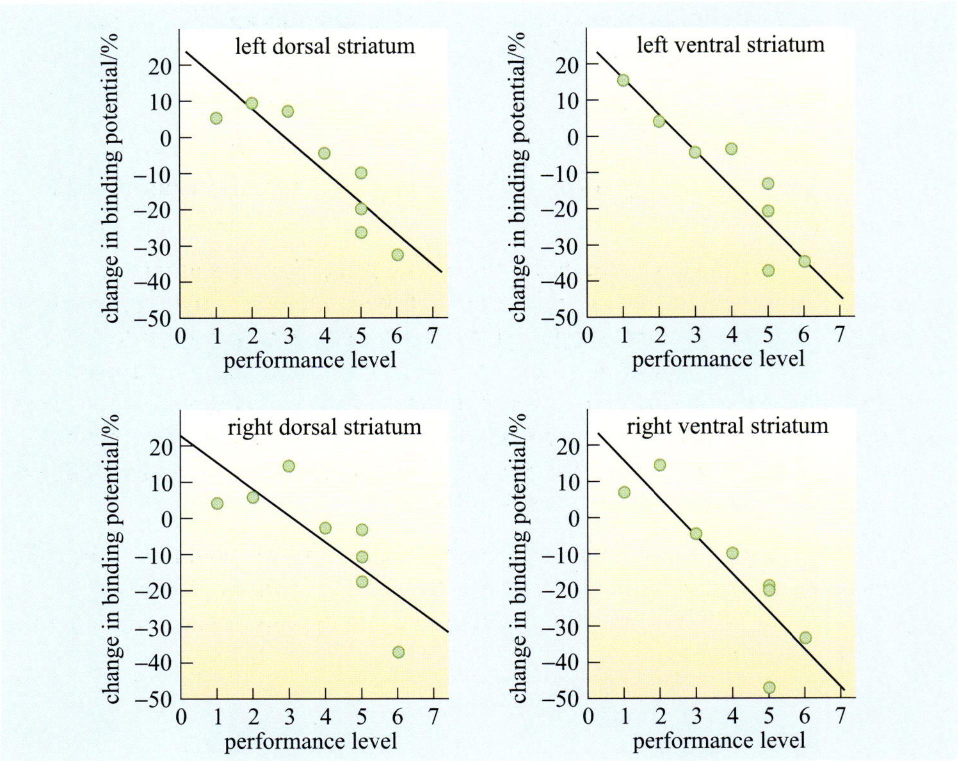

Figure 1.21 Percentage change in binding between task and baseline condition as a function of performance level for the eight participants.

Although much more work remains to be done, this result raises the possibility that DA activation is the biological basis of all addictive activities, whether drug related or non-drug related.

1.4.6 Trying to develop a theory of addiction

Biological psychologists try to give addiction research a broad theoretical basis by linking psychological phenomena to their roots in the nervous system. As an example of this, according to the highly influential theory of Terry Robinson and Kent Berridge, repeated exposure of the nervous system to addictive drugs causes what they term **incentive sensitization** to occur. This term describes a change in the properties of the motivational processes that underlie drug seeking and drug taking. The change is induced by the drug itself and is such that the neural processes come to induce an excessively high motivational 'pull' towards drug-related incentives, such as syringes or locations associated with drug taking.

So, the assumption of the theory is that sensitization can be triggered simply by the presence of the drug in the body. This induces changes in the structure of neurons, as shown in Figure 1.22.

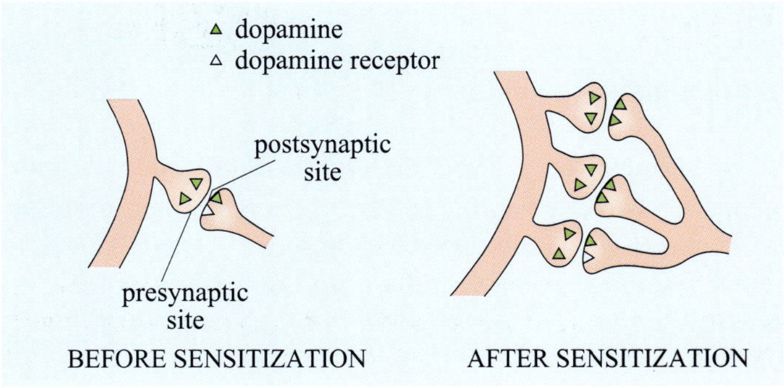

Figure 1.22 Changes at the level of dendritic spines, before and after sensitization. Note the expansion of contact area.

How could such sensitization be measured? Suppose that rats are divided into 3 groups as shown in Figure 1.23a.

- Group 1 are injected with the drug within a holding cage.
- Group 2 are injected with a control substance within a holding cage.
- Group 3 are given the injection of drug whilst in one arm of a T-maze (in this case, the white arm).

Subsequently, each group is held in the white arm of the T-maze and injected with drug (Figure 1.23b). The incentive value of the white arm is then measured (Figure 1.23c). Group 1 show a higher attraction to the white arm than do group 2. This shows that a prior injection of drug in a context different from the maze increases the incentive value of the arm of the maze that is subsequently associated with drug. However, group 3 show a stronger attraction to the injection side than do group 1. This shows the familiar power of the drug to lock into association with an external cue, in this case the white arm in part (a).

By extrapolation to the case of humans, Robinson and Berridge note that stimuli that in the past have been associated with taking drugs, such as the sight of a syringe or a region of town where drugs were purchased, trigger craving. This could in part reflect such sensitization.

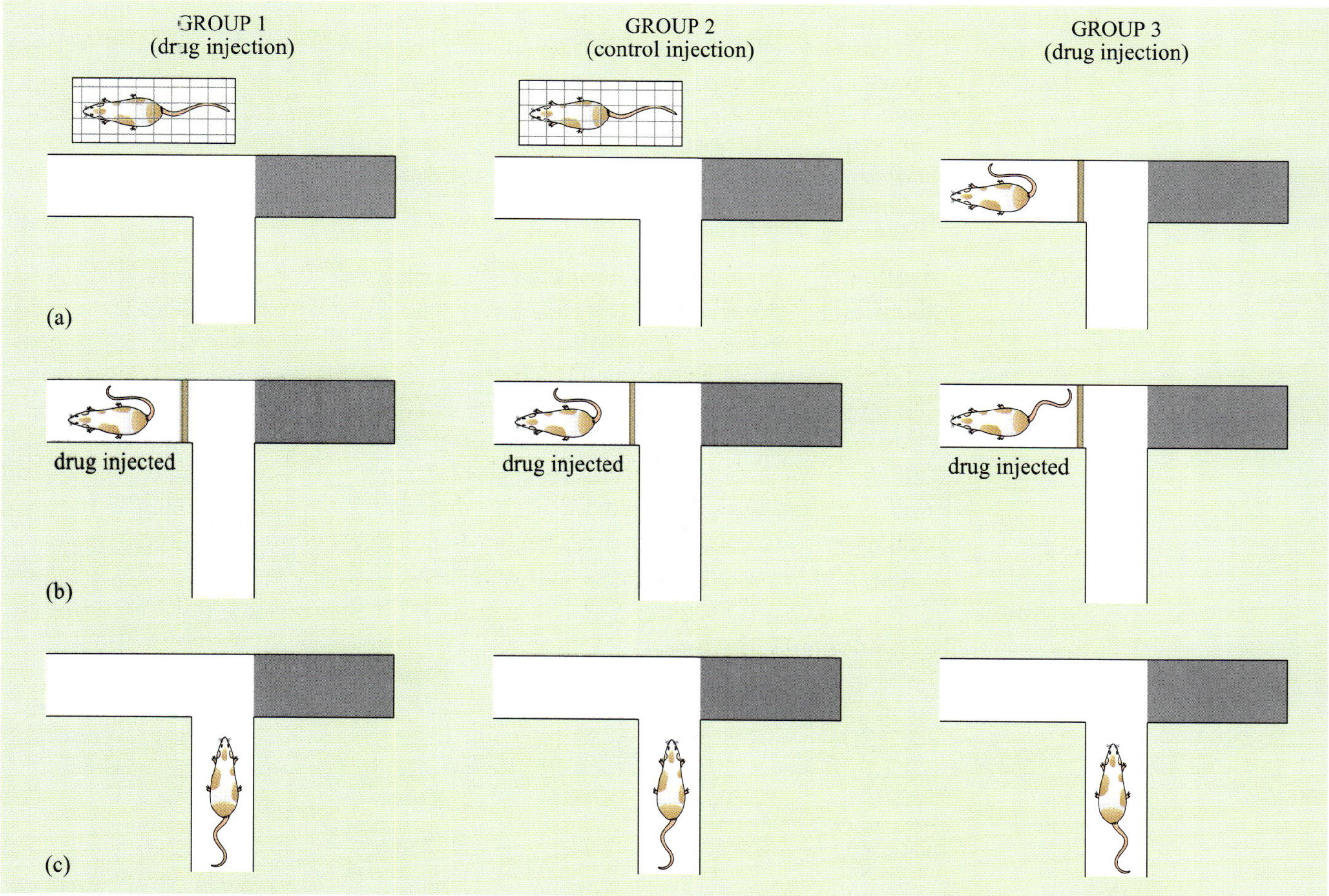

Figure 1.23 Experiment to demonstrate sensitization. (a) Group 1 are given prior injection of drug in an environment outside the T-maze; group 2 are given injection of control substance; group 3 are injected within one arm of the T-maze. (b) Each group is given an identical drug injection while in the white arm of the T-maze. (c) The rats in each group are put at the entrance to the T-maze and their preferences for the white and dark arms are measured.

To translate this to more everyday examples, could it be that, say, morphine taken for pain relief could increase the chances of subsequent addiction? If someone were inclined to take drugs for 'recreational' reasons in any case, such prior exposure might have a sensitizing effect. However, in reality, there is little danger of people who take drugs only for pain relief to lapse into addiction.

Towards a biologically based definition of addiction

Incentive sensitization can be defined independently of the behaviour that it is used to explain. The neural basis of such sensitization lies in the emergence of abnormalities in the nucleus accumbens and related neural structures. Abnormalities can be seen at the molecular level as well as at the level of the operation of whole neurons and the properties of the combinations of neurons that make up this system. There is a strengthening of excitatory synapses formed on the dopaminergic neurons. Changes in density of dendritic spines are observed and there is an increased postsynaptic density of DA receptors as a result of such sensitization (Figure 1.22). There is an increased ability of various drugs described as addictive to increase the release of DA in the nucleus accumbens.

- This is similar to what process you met earlier in the course?
- Long-term potentiation (Book 5, Section 1.7).

According to Robinson and Berridge, these changes represent the biological basis of the move to compulsive use of a drug. The changes at a neural level persist for years following the cessation of drug taking. Thereby, they produce a risk factor for relapse. This is the *wanting* part of the theory of Robinson and Berridge; incentive sensitization is associated with abnormally high wanting.

Wanting and liking

Section 1.1.3 drew a distinction between appetitive and consummatory aspects of motivation. A somewhat similar distinction emerges here: that between wanting and liking. Some initial contacts with drugs are described as euphoric, but many people report disliking their first experience of a drug such as alcohol, opiates or nicotine. Yet they still seek to repeat the experience. Robinson and Berridge believe that this is due in part to abnormal sensitization of the incentive system. A description of the underlying process of liking is also a part of the theory. Robinson and Berridge argue that as drugs are repeatedly taken, a fracture line between wanting and liking can appear (Figure 1.24). Initially, any hedonic effects of drugs will increase the strength of the wanting process. However, there is no one-to-one link between the strength of wanting and liking. Rather, as drugs are taken more and more, so wanting normally increases but paradoxically the pleasure derived from drugs ('liking') can decrease. From their own subjective experience, heroin addicts often describe such a dissociation.

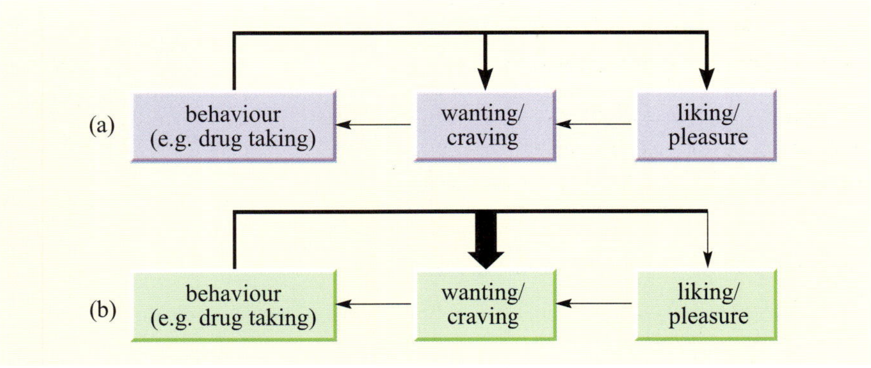

Figure 1.24 Representation of wanting and liking (a) initially and (b) following repeated experience.

Alas, according to incentive sensitization theory, addicts of hard drugs would seem to have everything going against them. Not only will their target drug trigger sensitization but so too might any alcohol and nicotine that they take. These can cause a cross-sensitization so that each drug will increase the craving for the others. There is evidence to suggest that nicotine is a so-called gateway drug to taking hard drugs. It is possible to see why this might be in terms of a sensitization of dopaminergic pathways by nicotine. The hard drug arrives at a system already sensitized. As if this were not enough, stress is also known to increase sensitization, hence contributing yet one more factor in the downward spiral. Why some users of hard drugs retain control is an interesting question. Such factors as differences in stress levels and alternative sources of obtaining reward come to mind.

We do not need to look to so-called hard drugs to find examples of the fracture line between wanting and liking. Nicotine is a notoriously difficult drug to give up and is known to trigger incentive sensitization. Wanting increases with exposure. People being treated for cancer and limb amputations as a result of tobacco use still continue, in many cases, to smoke. In one study, addicts of hard drugs undergoing therapy for this addiction ranked their parallel addiction to nicotine as being more difficult to break than that to the hard drug. Yet surely few would describe the effects of nicotine in such terms as a quite overwhelming pleasure or euphoria ('hedonism'), the strength of which escalates over time.

The theory appears to apply well to drug addiction. Whether it might be adapted to account for non-chemical addictions is a subject being studied.

Summary of Section 1.4

Attempts to define the term addiction have not brought complete agreement. The term embraces several possible criteria: craving, withdrawal symptoms, tolerance and disruption to life, and has been applied to both drug-related and some non-drug-related activities. Activation of dopaminergic pathways appears to be present in all activities that are described as addictive. In addition, opioidergic pathways are involved. An attempt to present a general theory of addiction was based on the notion of 'incentive sensitization' and refers to changes that occur in DA pathways as a result of exposure to drugs.

1.5 Final word and conclusion

The chapter has looked at some examples of motivation and has considered their common features and differences. In each case, it was shown where subjective evidence (such as a rating of palatability, a feeling of sexual desire, or a report of drug craving) and objective evidence (levels of neurotransmitter and hormones) need to be taken into account in providing an explanation. Craving was discussed mainly in the context of drugs but it also applies to other motivations. Cravings for food are increased by the sight or smell of the food or even by imagining the food.

Some motivations, such as those directed to food and water, form an integral part of homeostasis and correspondingly can be understood in terms of function. Sexual motivation is, of course, also explicable in terms of function. At base it appears not to be associated with homeostasis.

Not surprisingly, the motivation underlying addictive activities such as drug taking would appear not to fit functional explanations in any obvious way. What seems to happen is that drugs interact with brain processes that evolved to serve conventional motivations. It is surely not coincidence that dopaminergic and opioidergic neurotransmission featured both in the discussion of conventional motivations, i.e. feeding and sex, as well as drug taking. Not only do drugs interact with conventional motivational processes but they can usurp (or 'highjack') control from such conventional motivations. Another metaphor that could be useful is that they are *parasitic upon* the host motivational processes. Thus, in the competition for control of behaviour, thoughts of drugs can come to dominate conscious awareness and actions directed to obtaining drugs can dominate behaviour. Whereas the pull of, for example, nicotine-related cues appears to operate via the same mechanism as natural incentives such as food and sex, there is an important difference. Natural rewards, for instance a particular food, induce relatively long-term satiety. By contrast, apart from nausea or lack of availability, there is often rather little in the way of restraint corresponding to drugs. The 'two packs a day' smoker bears witness to this. According to the incentive sensitization theory, the presence of drugs causes changes within the structure of neural systems underlying motivation such as to give a bias towards engaging drug-related motivation.

The chapter has shown the ubiquitous role of conditioning in the expression of motivations in behaviour. In the case of feeding, sex and drug taking, cues that in the past were paired with the activity come to acquire motivational potential. Their presence plays a role in the future triggering of motivation.

Though not excluding a role for many other neurochemicals in motivation, the chapter has emphasized that of DA and opioids. DA has more to do with the organization of the appetitive ('seeking') phase of behaviour, whereas opioids play a role in the consequences of behaviour, such as computation of the palatability of food. Research currently in progress is directed to seeing whether the explanation of motivation and addiction in these terms can be extended to non-chemical addictions such as shopping, gambling and video games.

Although, for convenience, motivations have been discussed in separate sections, there are important interactions between them and insight can be gained by looking at their interdependence. This is what might be expected from the observation that certain common neurochemicals are employed throughout. In rodents, there exists an association between liking of sweet tastes and proneness to self-administer drugs. In humans, there is a correlation between a fondness for sweets and a proneness to drug taking. Addiction treatment programmes recommend sweets as a means of reducing craving for drugs.

Learning outcomes for Chapter 1

After studying this chapter, you should be able to:

1.1 Recognize definitions and applications of each of the terms printed in **bold** in the text.

1.2 Relate motivation to homeostasis and learning.

1.3 Describe some of the biological bases of motivation and link these to behaviour.

1.4 Describe the problems of designing experiments in the area of motivation.

1.5 Compare and contrast motivations.

1.6 Give an account of the problems associated with defining addiction and show the relevance of biological psychology to gaining insight.

1.7 Relate functional and causal explanations in the context of motivation.

Questions for Chapter 1

Question 1.1 *(Learning outcome 1.2)*

How is the principle of homeostasis illustrated by each of the following?

(a) In the case of the reaction to a concentrated sodium chloride solution, the move of taste reactivity in a positive direction following sodium depletion.

(b) In the case of the reaction to a sugar solution, the move of taste reactivity in a negative direction following taste-aversion conditioning.

Question 1.2 *(Learning outcomes 1.3 and 1.4)*

Section 1.4.6 described an experiment in which a rat is placed in a distinctive arm of a T-maze.

(a) Describe this experiment in such a way that the terms 'incentive' and 'classical conditioning' are made clear.

(b) Why is it necessary to counterbalance drug injections between black and white sides?

Question 1.3 *(Learning outcome 1.4)*

In the experiment shown in Figure 1.4, why were the bowls changed even in the condition where the same diet was given throughout?

Question 1.4 *(Learning outcomes 1.5 and 1.7)*

Why was it claimed that drug taking does not 'make sense' from a functional perspective 'in any obvious way'? Why the qualification 'in any obvious way'?

Question 1.5 *(Learning outcome 1.6)*

It used to be argued that craving is a purely subjective phenomenon. How have advances in technology forced us to qualify such a claim?

CHAPTER 2

EMOTION

2.1 Introduction

Emotions! Here, is a topic that many people consider should be central to understanding much of human behaviour, for throwing light on our happiness and on our miseries. The study of emotion has surely been fundamental to psychology from its very beginnings. Surprisingly, until recently, emotion research had a relatively minor and peripheral role in psychology. Emotional reactions have been more intensively studied from a biological standpoint, such as understanding the body's physiological responses to stress (Book 1, Section 3.5.1). In Book 6 Section 1.1.1, we considered the term 'motivation' and how we speak of someone being, for example, motivated by hunger, fear or greed. In this chapter we will turn the emphasis towards understanding these and other emotions, and look at the close links between research into emotions and into motivation.

- ◆ What is the scientific term that refers to the experience of pleasure or pain?
- ◆ Hedonics. This term was introduced in Sections 1.1.1, 1.2.4 and 1.4.6. It refers to the distinction, and sometimes dissociation, between liking (hedonics) and wanting (motivation).

Emotions are feelings that are familiar to us all and, starting from the cry of a newborn baby, accompany us in all their complexity and variety throughout our lives. Nevertheless, pick up any text on the subject, immerse yourself in the works of poets, read discussions of philosophers or anthropologists, and the dominant message that emerges is that, although they are universally experienced, we are sorely taxed when attempting to define clearly what we mean by emotions.

Emotions have many facets, and emotion researchers differ in the emphasis they place on the different aspects. They may study overt expression of emotion as revealed by behaviour, the mental state or 'feeling' of emotion as revealed by language, the internal physiological processes and hormonal responses (such as those involved in 'fight or flight' (Book 1, Box 3.3)), or brain areas concerned with different types of emotional processing. You will find it helpful to keep these distinctions in mind as you proceed through this chapter. Thus, there is no clear consensus on a definition of emotion, and researchers study different aspects, such as:

- behaviours (including facial expressions and 'body language')
- feelings (conscious awareness)
- physiological responses
- brain structure and function (including non-conscious processes).

This chapter will highlight some of the areas covered by emotion research. We will consider the universality, features and function of emotions, some of the brain structures implicated, and briefly reflect on emotional disorders.

2.2 Previous neglect of emotion research

- When, considering your everyday life, do you think that emotions are generally a hindrance or a help?
- It is not always easy to decide, but both can be true. Emotions can interrupt and interfere with ongoing tasks, but many a task would never be started without the prospect of the pleasure of success or the discomfort of failure and rejection. An emotional outburst of anger or distress may sometimes make some circumstances worse, but interrupting your routine and rapidly fleeing might be a lifesaver if you are confronted with a dangerous situation.

Many cultures value rational behaviour, and people in such cultures like to think of themselves as operating in a logical manner. When aroused by emotion, behaviour elicited in the 'heat of the moment' can be regretted on later reflection. Frequently, the failure to control such behaviour is labelled as a sign of weakness or a lack of maturity. It is emotion's ability to disrupt and interfere with ongoing tasks and thoughts that have given it a bad name. The benefits of both negative and positive emotions, and their possible functions in the course of evolution, have until recently been downplayed or overlooked.

Charles Darwin wrote perhaps the first book on the biological psychology of emotions, *The Expression of the Emotions in Man and Animals* (Darwin, 1872). He proposed that emotions and emotional expressions had become refined through natural selection and were therefore an advantage for our ancestors, but he assumed their usefulness was now outlived in humans. Thus he assumed that emotional expressions now occur in adult humans 'though they may not … be of the least use'. Some physical characteristics of emotions, such as our hair standing on end during fear or anger, show parallels in other mammals. This can have the dramatic effect of making other animals look larger (Figure 2.1) and potentially intimidating the aggressor. Darwin would be correct, of course, in noting that a similar reaction has a rather limited function in humans.

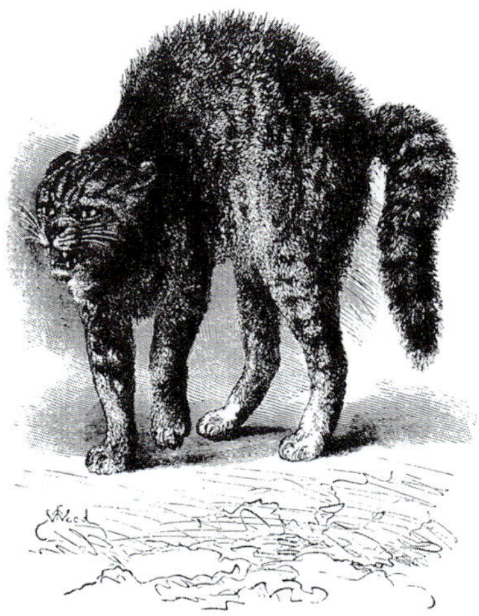

Figure 2.1 Animals use a range of methods to display emotion. A cat uses body signals (e.g. raised back), facial expression (e.g. lips retracted to expose teeth) and hair standing on end as an aggressive display in the face of threat.

For Darwin, emotions were a bit like vestigial parts of the body, such as the appendix in the digestive system that is an evolutionary hangover from times when it did have a useful function. Emotions seemed to hint at animal or infantile origins, but did not prompt him to search for any current function. Indeed, at least since Plato (375 BC), many Western thinkers have viewed emotions as impediments to rational thought or, at best, harmless asides.

Until recently, emotions have not been regarded as worthy of serious scientific consideration in psychology, unlike other topics such as perception, language, thinking and learning. Part of this neglect is that emotions were, and to some extent still are, often considered to be childish, destructive and best suppressed by upright, virtuous citizens. This view was especially true in Darwin's day. Little wonder he felt that:

> Our descent, then, is the origin of our evil passion!! – The Devil under form of baboon is our grandfather.
>
> (Darwin, cited in Oatley and Jenkins, 1996, p. 2)

2.3 Universality of emotions

Despite Darwin's dismissive attitude towards the utility of emotion in humans, he was interested in the universality of their expression. From his travels around the world, careful studies of emotional expressions in his own children and inmates in mental asylums, as well as observations of other cultures by missionaries, he concluded that emotional expressions were universal (Figure 2.2). He noted that people from different cultures convey their emotions with the same facial expressions, even though local languages and customs differ widely. A smile is understood the world over. Certain emotions, such as anger, sadness, fear, affection, pleasure and pain seemed to Darwin to be universal and inherited. Human emotional expression is not confined to the face – body movement, posture, tone of voice and skin colour can all contribute. Even without words, this rich and varied repertoire can convey a great deal of information about a person's emotional status. Emotional expressions are at least partially automatic since, as Figure 2.3 shows, they are performed by people when they are on the telephone, even though they cannot be seen by whoever is on the other end of the line. It has been suggested that these expressions help the linguistic fluency of the speaker. Try giving complex directions to somewhere without moving your body, especially your hands. Does this make it more difficult to give the directions?

Pause for a moment and bring to mind a time when you felt very angry and another occasion when you felt very happy.

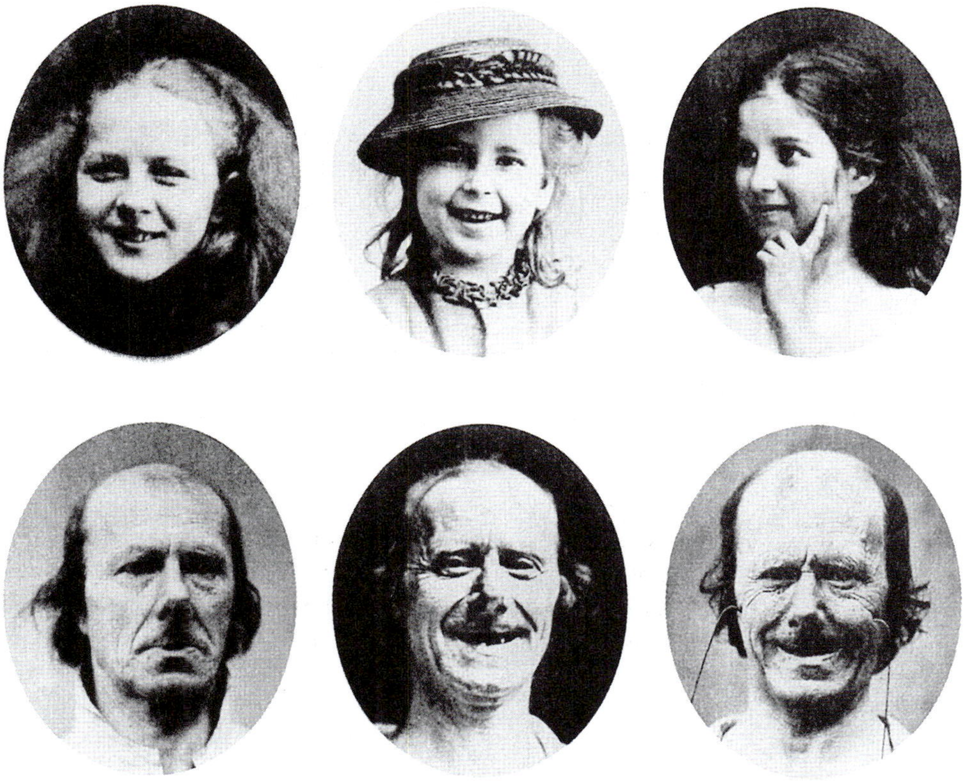

Figure 2.2 A range of human facial expressions taken from Darwin's book *The Expressions of the Emotions in Man and Animals*.

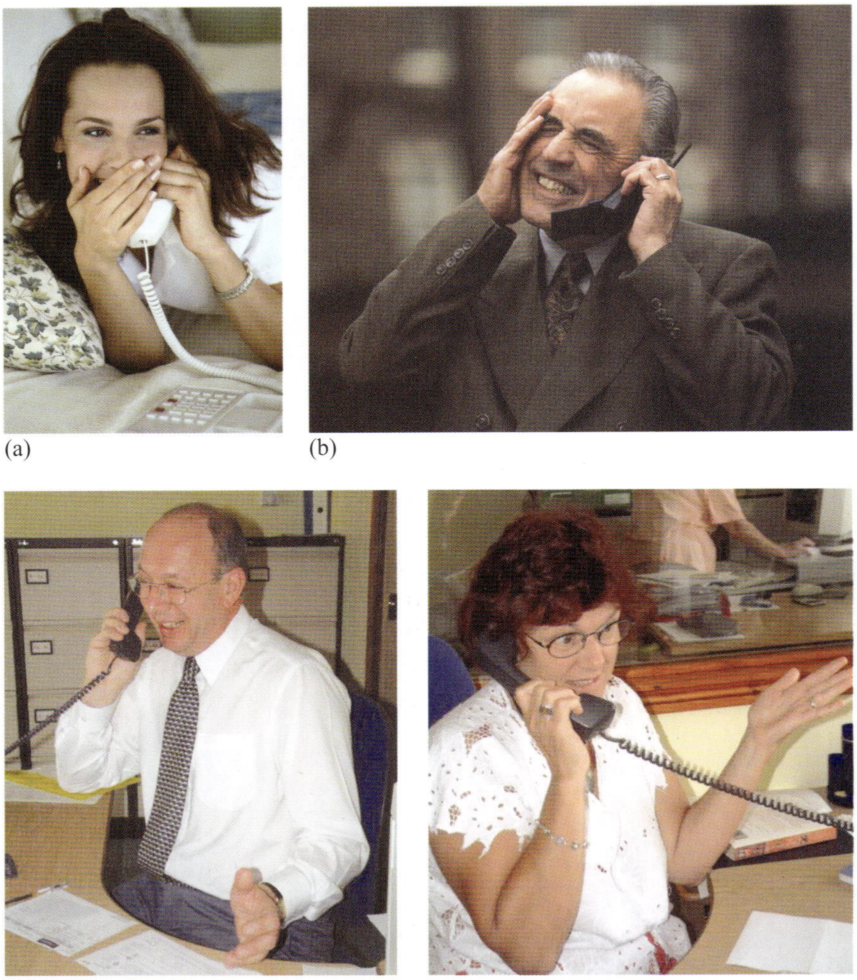

(a) (b) (c) (d)

Figure 2.3 Humans continue to perform a range of body expressions, such as in these examples of telephone conversations, even when they cannot be communicated to the person at the other end. Perhaps, however, they help the linguistic fluency of the speaker.

Did you find that your facial muscles moved first into a slight frown and then into a smile? Many people find that this does happen, illustrating that emotional expressions are not generated consciously for the purpose of communicating emotional information to others.

- Can you think of another type of situation when we become particularly aware of how automatic our emotional expressions can be?
- One example is when we try to disguise emotions, whether out of politeness or deceit. It is hard to suppress entirely all indications of our emotions. The successful control of facial expression is often accompanied by giveaway cues in body language or tone of voice.

In humans, differences in cultures and languages lead to huge variations in behaviour and it has sometimes been speculated that emotional expressions could be learnt as part of the socialization process and may therefore differ across cultures. In other animals, the biological origins of emotion expression are rarely disputed and many complex expressions of emotion can be seen, indicated by features such as vocalizations, body posture, facial expression, skin colour or special odours such as pheromones. Figure 2.4 shows a dog in an aggressive and a submissive posture. Notice that raising or lowering the body hair is a feature that adds to the impact of the dog's display.

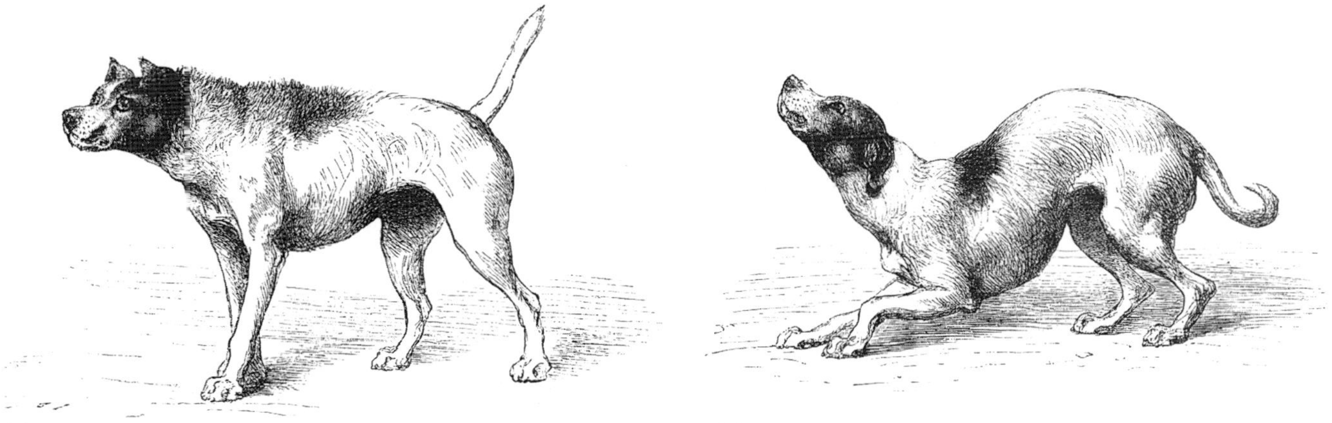

(a) (b)

Figure 2.4 Two opposite emotions in a dog: (a) aggression and (b) submission. Notice how elements of the submissive posture seem 'opposite' to those in the aggressive one, e.g. tail, shoulder and hackles are raised in aggression but lowered in appeasement.

If humans share emotional experiences and can readily recognize emotional expressions worldwide, then this could be evidence pointing towards the biological origins of emotional expressions. From his descriptive studies, Darwin assumed this universality, and this conclusion has also been reached in more recent and carefully controlled experiments. Probably the best known series of experiments was carried out by Paul Ekman and his collaborators (Ekman and Friesen, 1986; 1988). They took photographs of North Americans displaying a range of emotion expressions. These were shown to different tribes people, including the New Guinea Fore people who at the time had had minimal contact with Western society. In turn, he photographed responses to emotional situations in these peoples, which were later judged by North Americans. The conclusion was that both recognition and expression of emotions were shared across cultures, at least for the six emotions that he considered 'basic': happiness, surprise, sadness, anger, fear and disgust. Although all these emotions seemed 'basic', they were not equally easy to recognize. Happiness was always the easiest to recognize, with some confusion occurring between the negative emotions which were more difficult to identify precisely. Surprise and fear produced the most uncertainty. There is now a large body of research supporting the pancultural nature of the recognition of expressions and of the way that expressions are produced (from recordings of facial muscle activity).

◆ What might the pictures in Figure 2.5, which are of a child blind from birth, tell us about how facial expressions are acquired?

◆ Blind children, who could never have learnt by example, produce spontaneous facial expressions. This lends further weight to the notion that facial expressions are inherited.

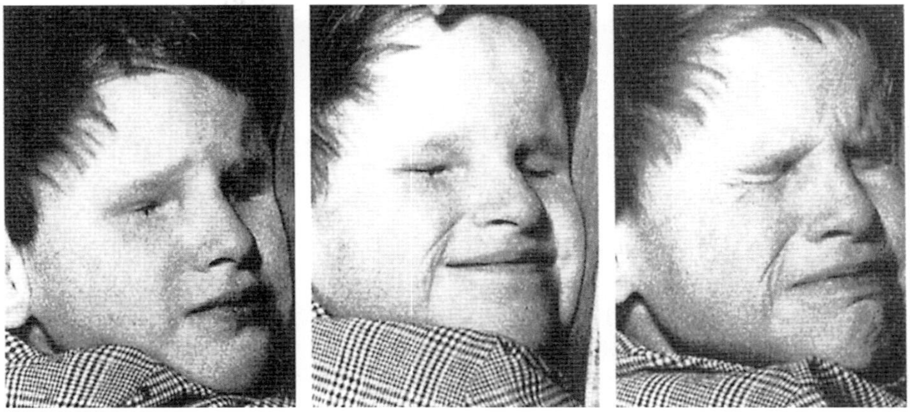

Figure 2.5 The facial expressions of a child blind from birth cannot have resulted from imitation.

2.3.1 Control of the expression of emotion

Some situations that trigger human emotions, such as the fear evoked by encountering a large predator, seem universal. However, without doubt there are cultural and individual differences in what elicits a particular emotion. These differences extend also to the attempts of individuals to control emotional expression and, presumably, to the acquisition of the ability to achieve this control. For instance, in many non-Western cultures there is much more emphasis on the social group, with the needs of the individual being secondary, whereas the reverse is predominantly found in Europe and North America. There is a marked contrast in these cultures between the rights and responsibilities of individuals towards society. In Japan, for example, it is thought to be highly inappropriate to express anger towards relations or colleagues (those within your social group) whilst anger between North Americans who know and like each other is common and in many situations generally accepted. An outward display of happiness is considered inappropriate at a Japanese wedding: a serious attitude is expected (Figure 2.6a). An outward display of sadness may be considered impolite in Japan: a slight smile is expected. This would be considered rather ominous in other societies, for example British wedding guests smile at weddings (Figure 2.6b) but are serious at funerals (Figure 2.6c). The culturally polite control of emotion in Japan, such as at the death of a loved one, could easily be misinterpreted as a lack of feeling and contrasts starkly with the very public wailing displayed at, for example, a Palestinian funeral (Figure 2.6d). Children take time to learn these unwritten rules and to control their emotional expressions, so they often break the local social codes.

From research, Ekman and Friesen suggest that it is the expression rather than the experience of emotion that varies with culture. Japanese and American participants, either alone or in the presence of others, were secretly videoed watching unpleasant film clips, such as nasal surgery. When alone, the expressions of fear and disgust were equally prevalent, but with others present in the room the emotional expressions of the Japanese were greatly inhibited – they covered up their feelings by smiling instead. Revealingly, slow-motion replay of the videos suggested fleeting beginnings of fear and disgust expressions were rapidly overlaid by social smiling. Social control of expressions results in the rapid inhibition, not the elimination, of their display.

Summary of Sections 2.2–2.3

Emotion research covers distinct aspects of emotion such as feeling states, physiological responses and behaviour. Despite a range of cultural differences in the accepted display of emotions in humans, researchers assume that there are a number of so-called basic emotions that appear to be universal and biologically determined.

2.4 Locating basic emotions in the brain

From Section 2.3, you will have noted that there seems to be agreement that some 'basic', and thus universal, emotions exist. Although there is variation among researchers, the number of these basic emotions is assumed to be around six, corresponding, more or less, with the range of facial expressions originally identified by Darwin. Some minor debate surrounds the appropriate names for them; for instance, should we designate 'happiness' as the universal positive

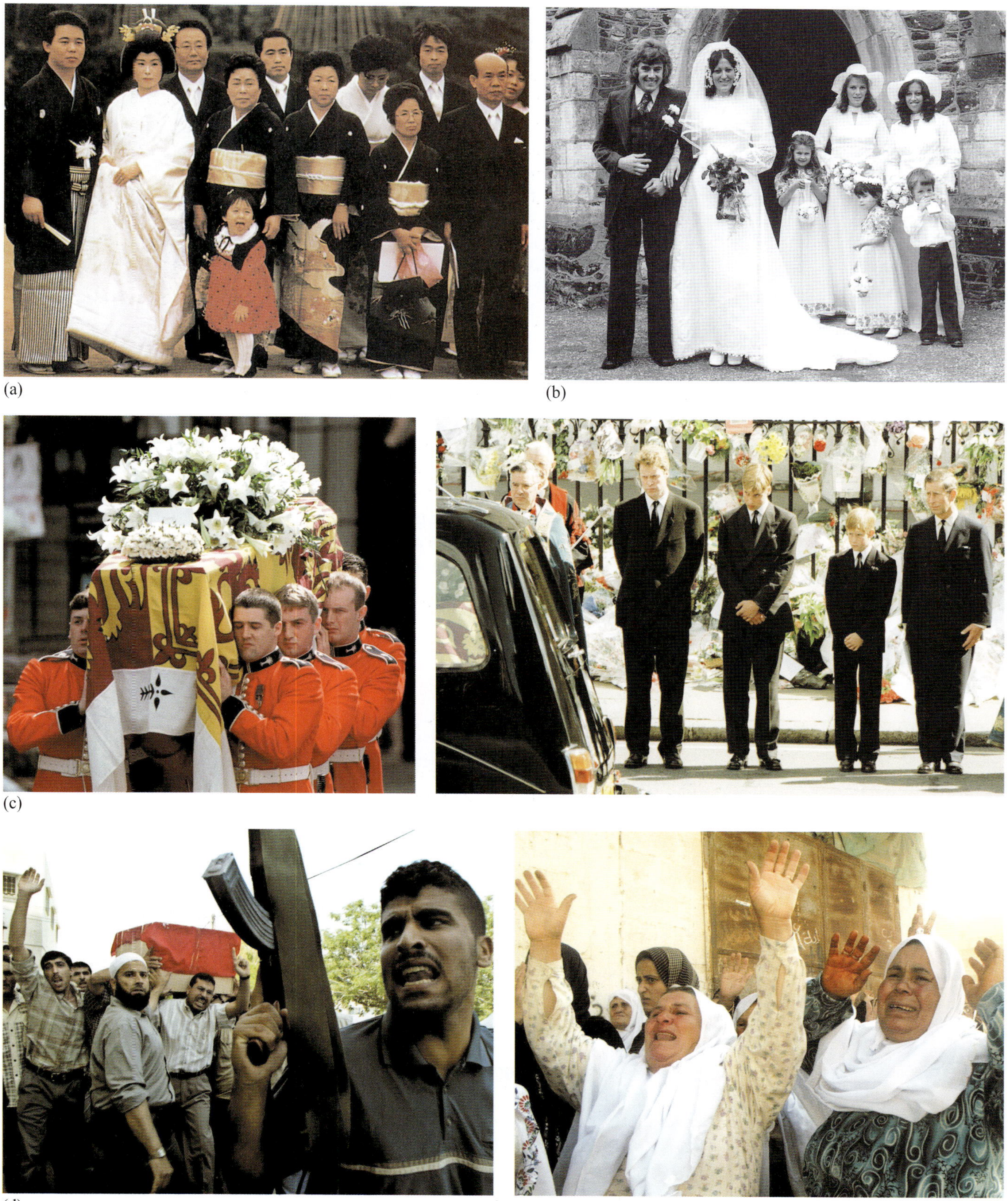

Figure 2.6 The socially appropriate display of emotions differs between cultures. (a) At a wedding in Japan, a serious expression might be expected whereas in Britain (b) the wedding guests smile more conspicuously. At a funeral in Europe or North America it may be appropriate to be quiet and solemn, as shown in the images taken at the funeral of Princess Diana (c), or cry out and wail with grief (d), depending on the culture. Children take time to learn these unwritten rules.

emotion or is this a mood and 'joy' the term appropriate for describing an emotion? (Evans, 2001). Most researchers would agree to a list including:

happiness	sadness	anger
fear	surprise	disgust

What is the evidence for the biological underpinnings of these distinctions? Are different brain areas and neural pathways associated with each basic emotion? As may become apparent as you read on, there has been marked inequality in research effort across the range of emotions. The emphasis below largely reflects this imbalance, for instance 'surprise' is rarely studied. As we will be referring to the brain areas involved in emotions in this section, you may want to revisit Book 1, Section 3.4 or the multimedia package *Exploring the Brain* to remind yourself of the locations of the hippocampus, amygdala, and hypothalamus. You may recall that the amygdala and hippocampus form part of the limbic system which is closely linked with the hypothalamus.

These areas are deep within the brain and their involvement in emotion has been known for a long time. In the 1930s, Kluver and Bucy discovered that removal of the temporal lobes (including the amygdala and parts of the hippocampus) had a dramatic effect on emotional responses in monkeys. The monkeys, who prior to the intervention were fearful and sometimes aggressive, were now quite fearless and calm. They seemed to see but not to recognize the (emotional) meaning of common objects. A hungry monkey would normally quickly identify familiar food by sight, making a beeline for it and hastily cramming it into its mouth. However, after the removal of the temporal lobes, this directed, purposeful looking behaviour was lost. Instead, the monkeys would examine anything they came across, testing each item in their mouths and then eating it if it was food. In addition, whereas formerly they would have been very wary of natural enemies, such as snakes, they would now make indiscriminate approaches to anything in their environment, and even the experience of being attacked failed to make them more cautious. This constellation of symptoms has become known as the **Kluver–Bucy syndrome**, and appears to consist of a separation between the sensory processing of stimuli and the attribution of affective value, or emotional significance, to them. Many of these characteristics have also been seen in humans unfortunate enough to have suffered temporal lobe damage. In addition to the visual recognition problems, they report 'flattened' or diminished emotional experiences.

These early studies removed relatively large areas of the brain, so research effort has continued in the quest to localize more specific brain areas responsible for specific emotional experiences and responses. In particular, investigations have tried to identify whether different brain areas are involved in different basic emotions. In this section, we consider evidence from brain damage, lesions and stimulation and then in Section 2.5 we reflect on evidence from brain imaging.

2.4.1 Anger and aggression

Early studies involving massive damage to the cerebral hemispheres of cats or dogs resulted in animals that would overreact and go into a state of 'violent rage' at the slightest provocation – snarling, bearing teeth, hissing, flattening ears, and so on. Previously docile animals would react this way when, for instance, they were merely stroked on the back, which they had previously showed signs of enjoying. The state that was invoked was called 'sham rage' because, although giving strong outward displays of threat and aggression, attack rarely followed, and the 'rage' dissipated rather rapidly. Further studies suggested that it was the posterior region of the hypothalamus that was vital for this rage response. Using electrical stimulation through implanted electrodes, Hess (1920s), Flynn (1960s) and others were able to evoke either aggressive displays or outright attack by placing electrodes within the medial and lateral areas respectively of the hypothalamus. Because different brain areas are involved, does this mean there is more than one type of aggressive emotion? The answer is yes. In the studies above, for instance, a distinction was made between two types of aggression:

- *threat* aggression, such as when two cats aggressively arch their backs, hiss, spit and threaten to, or actually, attack each other;
- *predatory* aggression, such as when a cat stealthily approaches a prey animal and makes a rapid and silent attack to kill.

This distinction serves as a reminder that emotions are complex, and that placing them under the headings of six 'basic' emotions is bound to be a gross oversimplification.

One area of the brain, the amygdala, is particularly important for many emotions, including aggression. Removing the amygdala of high-ranking monkeys results in a decrease in aggression. The animals become very submissive and rapidly slip down to a low-ranking status. Additional evidence that the amygdala is involved in aggression comes from electrical stimulation of different areas of the amygdala that can either inhibit or induce aggression, depending on the location. In some humans with anger problems, their very violent behaviour has been thought to be triggered by seizures activating the amygdala. Recognizing that aggression can be reduced by brain operations in animals, some people have had their amygdala surgically removed. This type of operation, termed **psychosurgery**, was relatively common in the early part of the 20th century, particularly in the USA (for example, see Box 2.1 on frontal lobotomy). Although frequently accompanied by disastrous side effects, clinical reports suggest that amygdala removal successfully reduced aggressive antisocial behaviour, and in addition increased the ability to concentrate. However, these benefits come at a cost. Amygdala damage in humans is associated with a general reduction in emotionality as well as a reduced (or absent) ability to recognize emotion in others. (This relates to a range of emotions, not just fear and aggression, as we shall explore below.) Failing to recognize or anticipate emotion in others is socially extremely handicapping and the inappropriate behaviour that results can be very disrupting to social bonds.

Attempts to study anger and aggression in humans using brain-imaging techniques are relatively few. When participants were asked to view facial expressions showing anger then the amygdala seemed to be activated, but in other studies when participants were asked to recall personal past anger episodes the amygdala was not activated. Thus, as we considered at the beginning of this chapter, it seems important to make a distinction between different aspects of emotion. The areas of the brain involved in the feeling of emotion may contrast with those related to the recognition, induction or execution of emotion.

Box 2.1 Frontal lobotomy

Following the discoveries by Kluver, Bucy and others that the damage to the frontal cortex had effects on emotional behaviour, it was not long before those trying to treat emotionally disturbed humans targeted this area. Egas Moniz was the first to perform a prefrontal lobotomy on one of his patients, which was reported to be so successful that many others followed. In 1949, Moniz won a Nobel Prize for his work. (You may consider that it was poetic justice that by this time he had been shot by one of his lobotomized patients and was a paraplegic.)

A frightening array of techniques became standard for this operation. One technique known as 'ice pick psychosurgery' is shown in Figure 2.7. A knife was inserted through the top of the eye's orbit and the handle swung medially and laterally to destroy cells and interconnecting pathways. One of the advantages of this technique was that it left no obvious scar and was so simple it could even be performed in a physician's office.

Frontal lobotomy often reduced the patient's emotional suffering (particularly in cases of severe depression, anxiety and obsessive compulsive disorder). However, it had unfortunate side effects, such as a blunting of emotional responses, a reduction of social inhibitions, which led to inappropriate behaviours similar to those of Phineas Gage (Book 1, Section 1.1.4), and difficulty in making plans and working towards goals.

Treatment with this type of gross psychosurgery is now infrequent, mainly because of the development of drug therapy. However, some more focused microsurgery still takes place on some patients who fail to respond to drug treatment.

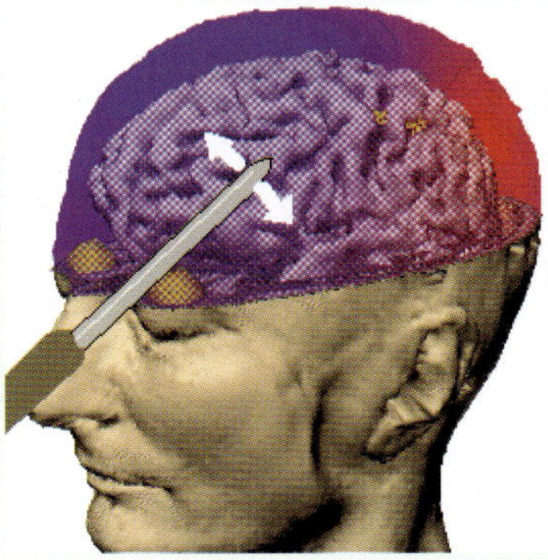

Figure 2.7 'Ice pick psychosurgery'. Arrows indicate movement of knife.

2.4.2 Fear

Damage to the amygdala alters aggressive responsiveness, but this area of the brain has been particularly implicated in fear and the control of fear responses. What do we mean here by fear responses? In Section 2.1 we saw that emotion has many aspects. A 'fear response' could include feelings of fear (we can only assess this response in humans who can tell us how they feel), behavioural changes (including fleeing, freezing, facial expressions of fear, and so on) and physiological changes (more about this later in the chapter). These are all associated with the activation of particular brain areas or pathways. One response to fear is the fear-potentiated startle response. When a loud noise is heard, we (and other animals) respond with a startle, in other words we jump and blink. (Other changes also take place such as a change in heart rate, but that is a slower response.) If we are afraid, then the startle response becomes exaggerated, we jump more noticeably and to a less-intense noise – this is the fear-potentiated startle, the extent to which the normal startle is intensified by fear. Lesions in the amygdala dramatically reduce fear responses, such as the fear-potentiated startle, and reduce or abolish conditioned fear. You have come across conditioned fear (classical conditioning in Book 5, Section 1.2.5), in which a conditioned response developed to a once neutral stimulus through repeated pairing with something unpleasant (e.g. electric shock). Activation of the amygdala greatly increases the startle response. Electrical stimulation of the amygdala in humans has reportedly led to anxiety and fear, and imaging studies indicate activation of this region when viewing fearful faces or pictures of threatening or frightening scenes.

- When a brain-imaging study shows the amygdala to be active in humans, could you conclude that the person is feeling fearful?
- Not necessarily. You may recall that pictures of fearful faces presented so briefly that they remain outside awareness can still give rise to activation of the amygdala in brain-imaging studies (Book 1, Section 4.3.2).

In line with the evidence of the involvement of the amygdala in fear, several human patients with damage to this structure have been found to have abnormal responses to fear stimuli, such as being unable to recognize both facial expressions (Figure 2.8) and vocalizations of fear. Another patient, known as S.M., studied by Adolphs and colleagues, was able to identify particular individuals from their photographs (this suggests that her vision and ability to detect subtle facial differences must have been normal). She could readily give the correct verbal label to happy, sad and disgust expressions, but was somewhat confused by angry faces. However, it was her responses to expressions of fear that were the most abnormal. She was very unlikely to identify this expression as being fear. In comparison with her accuracy for all other expressions, her performance for identifying fearful faces was notably impaired.

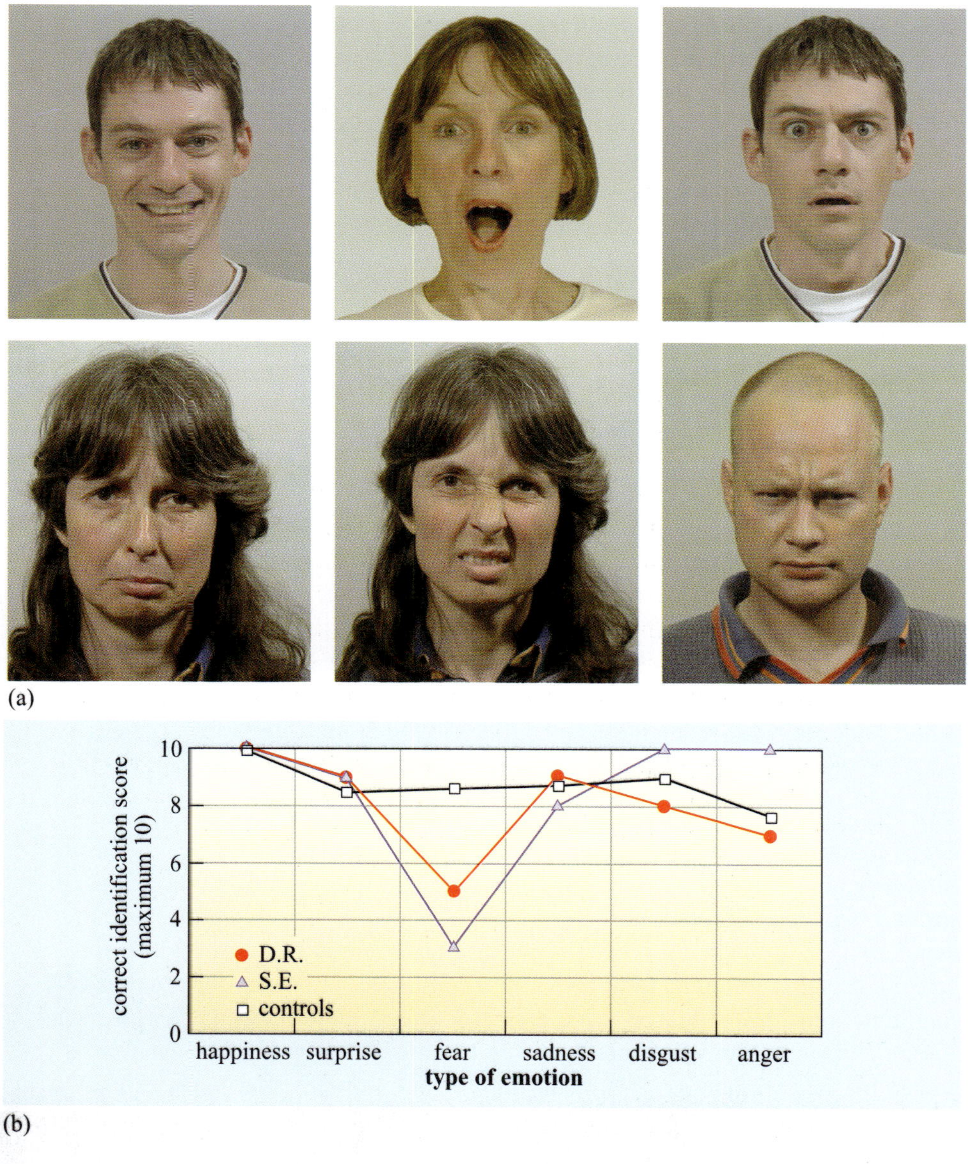

Figure 2.8 When patients with amygdala damage are asked to categorize facial expressions, such as those shown in (a), they have great difficulty with the emotion of fear, as can be seen in (b). (b) The performance of two such patients, known as S.E. and D.R., are plotted alongside a group of matched normal controls for comparison. Their task was to look at each expression and indicate which expression – happiness, surprise, fear, sadness, disgust or anger – was shown. As can be seen in the graph, the patients were very poor at giving the correct name to the fear expression, but they were quite good at all other emotions, especially happiness.

During fear conditioning, recordings can be taken that track the changing response of the amygdala as learning takes place. For instance, neurons in the amygdala can 'learn' to respond to stimuli associated with pain. In a situation in which two tones are presented, one paired with an unpleasant stimulus (such as mild electric shock) and the other one not, neurons originally insensitive to these initially neutral stimuli gradually become activated in response to the fear conditioned tone, but not to the benign tone (Book 5, Figure 1.26). Once the amygdala is activated, a fear response will be initiated (part of which is the increase in heart rate, and so on). The amygdala is not a primary location for memory storage, but it gives emotional content to memories. We will return to the amygdala in Section 2.5.1 and consider in more detail the pathways involving this structure.

- What type of learning is described in the above paragraph?
- This is a form of classical conditioning (Book 5, Section 1.2.1).

Just as with aggression, it is likely to be a gross oversimplification to assume that fear is a single entity. As an example, at least three different reactions to fear have been identified in infant monkeys: calling and cooing, freezing, and an agitated barking threat display. The infants were fearful because of being separated from their mothers and then being confronted with the approach of a stranger. That these three fear reactions were distinct is supported by the differential effects of drugs upon them. The calling and cooing behaviour decreased when opiate drugs were given, but increased in the presence of an opiate blocker (naloxone) whilst the other behaviours were unaffected by these drugs. Benzodiazepine drugs (diazapam) had no effect on cooing but decreased the other responses (freezing and barking) to an immediate threat such as the close approach of a stranger.

2.4.3 Happiness and pleasure

The role of opioids and the mesolimbic dopaminergic system in motivation and hedonics in relation to appetite and sexual behaviour should already be familiar to you (Sections 1.2.4 and 1.3).

- Which neurotransmitters seem to be associated with the feeling of pleasure?
- The opioids have a particular role in determining the hedonic value of a situation, whilst dopamine is more closely associated with the wanting aspect of motivation.

Just as researchers have explored brain areas associated with fear, anger and aggression, they have also attempted to locate centres involved in pleasure. In the 1950s, Olds and Milner implanted electrodes in the brains of rats to explore the effects of electrical stimulation in a variety of brain areas.

After the electrodes were implanted into a variety of brain sites, the rats were placed in Skinner boxes, but rather than rewarding lever-presses with food in the usual way, the rats were given a brief electrical stimulus directly to the brain. In certain brain sites (Figure 2.9), this resulted in rapid learning and persistent responding, so much so that the rats would often become so involved in lever-pressing that they shunned food and water, continuing until they were exhausted. The brain areas that produced these dramatic effects were dubbed 'pleasure centres'. Obviously, it would be helpful to be able to verify which sensations are evoked by such stimulation in humans but it is not normally feasible or ethical to

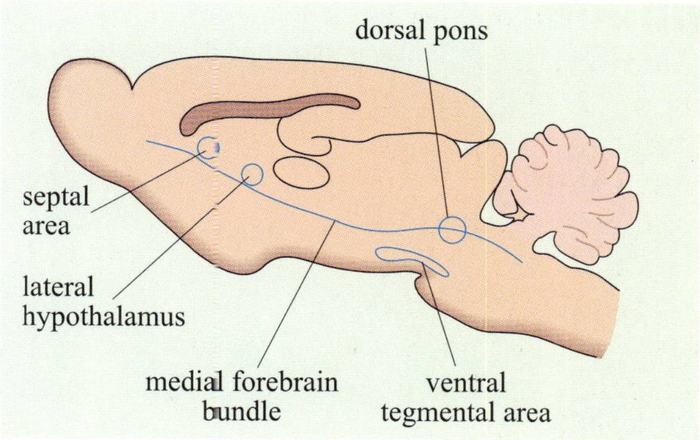

Figure 2.9 Sites of self-stimulation in the brain of the rat (blue). When electrodes are located in the marked areas, rats will work to receive electrical stimulation.

perform such studies. However, certain brain operations performed on humans, such as surgical treatment for severe epilepsy, require that the patient is alert throughout. During such procedures, electrical stimulation has sometimes evoked pleasurable feelings, suggesting that the term 'pleasure centre' might be appropriate. In some other procedures, however, when patients were able to self-stimulate, the brain site they chose did not give rise to pleasure. One patient had electrodes implanted in 17 brain sites and stimulation was applied to each separately. He reported feelings of pleasure from stimulation of the septal area and the midbrain tegmentum. Other mildly positive feelings were produced by stimulating areas in the amygdala and caudate nucleus, but the site he most frequently stimulated was in the medial thalamus. Here, the sensation reported was not of pleasure but of an irritable feeling. Stimulating this area produced the feeling that an important memory was about to be recalled. Repeated stimulation was reported as an insistent but futile attempt to bring the memory to mind, which ended in frustration.

- Can we be sure that the rats in Olds' and Milner's experiments were experiencing pleasure?

- No. We can only comment that they worked hard to repeat the stimulation, indicating that the stimulation motivated them to respond by pressing the lever. (You could call this 'wanting'.) The hedonic consequences of stimulation, however, cannot be assessed from their studies.

2.4.4 Disgust

When considering fear, we described someone suffering from brain damage that interfered with their ability to experience fear or to identify it in others, whilst other emotions were apparently normal. This same dissociation between different 'basic' emotions has been observed in people suffering from Huntington's disease or from damage to very specific brain regions. For these individuals, most emotional experiences seem normal except for that of disgust. In the facial recognition task mentioned earlier in Section 2.4.2, in which expressions of fear and anger were difficult for S.M. to identify, the performance of those with Huntington's disease or with brain lesions in the insula and putamen regions is normal except when presented with the disgust expression. Not only is this expression confused with other negative emotions in such a recognition task, but the experience, as well as the recognition of disgust, is also abnormal. This failure to be disgusted (when appropriate), and willingness to do things that others find disgusting, can be very distressing to close friends and relatives in social settings. Interestingly, in Huntington's disease, some changes in disgust sensitivity became detectable even before other, more characteristic, symptoms of the disease have emerged.

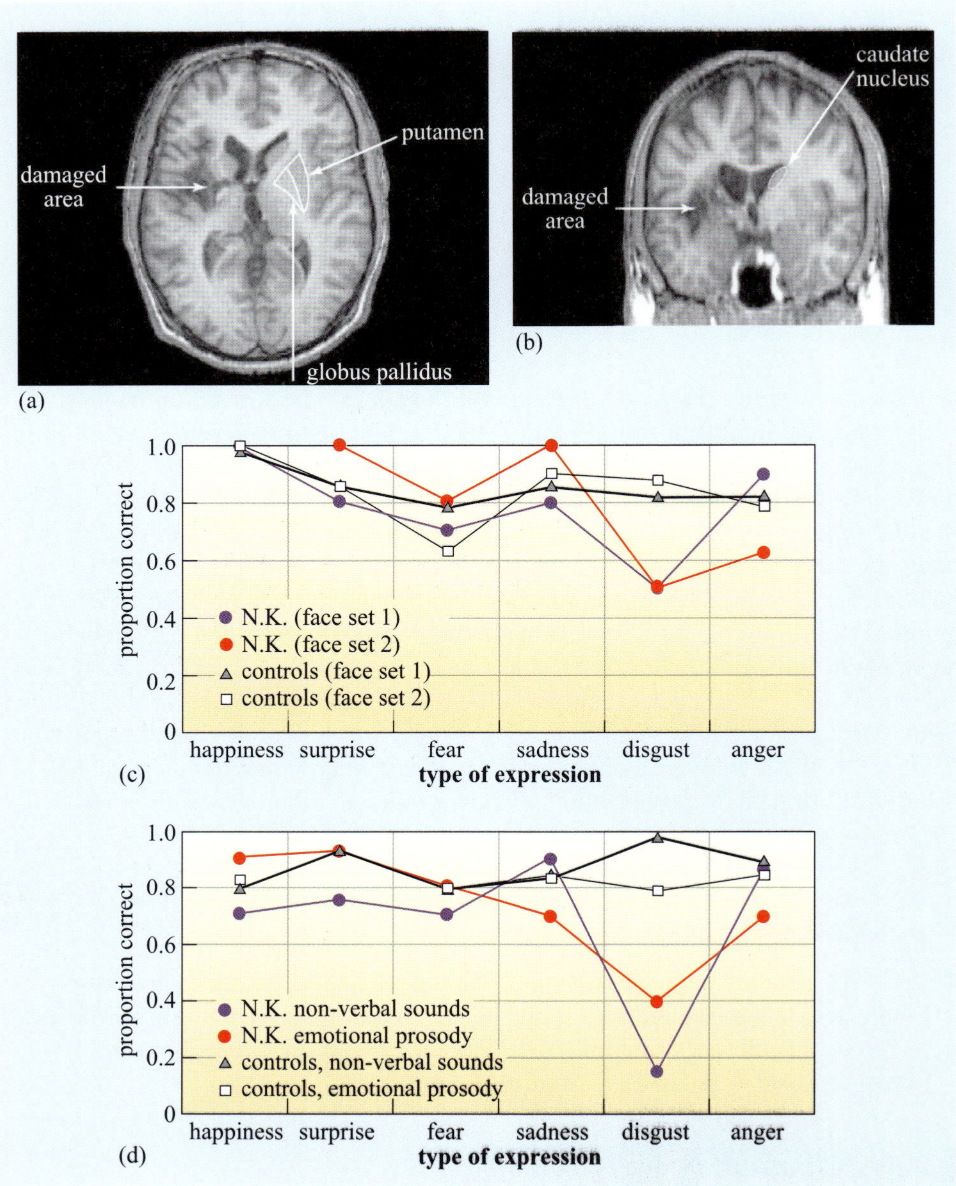

Figure 2.10 Magnetic resonance images: (a) an axial image, (b) a coronal image, showing brain damage to the left hemisphere after a stroke in a patient known as N.K. who, as a result, suffers impaired recognition of the emotion of disgust. The areas of damage are labelled. The equivalent undamaged areas are marked in the intact right hemisphere. (c) and (d) Graphs of the behavioural data showing N.K.'s ability to recognize emotions; (c) shows performance on a facial expression task similar to that shown in Figure 2.8 but using two separate sets of facial expressions. In addition, in (d), N.K. was tested on his ability to recognize non-verbal sounds of a range of emotions including disgust, and the non-verbal aspects of speaking that form part of the emotional communication when we speak. These are aspects such as tone of voice, loudness, stress and speed of speaking (called emotional prosody). In each case, the performance was compared with control participants matched in age and background. Notice that N.K.'s performance is very similar to that of the controls for all emotions except disgust. (No data are available for the emotional prosody control for surprise.)

Localized brain damage from injury or stroke can also result in selective impairment of the ability to experience and recognize the emotion of disgust, as demonstrated in Figure 2.10.

- Can you think of a reason why the participants in the study shown in Figure 2.10 were asked to categorize two different sets of facial expressions?

- One reason might be that the experimenters wanted to be sure that N.K.'s difficulty was not just caused by particular feature(s) of the faces forming one of the sets. Similar results were obtained with another set of individuals posing the range of emotion expressions. By repeating the task, the experimenters can be more confident that it is the expression of disgust that is causing difficulty for N.K. and not some aspect of the way this emotion is displayed by the individuals posing for one of the sets of photographs. The experimenters were trying to ensure that their results were not caused by an extraneous variable (Book 2, Section 1.2.3).

Summary of Section 2.4

The amygdala is vital for processing emotion and, when damaged, the recognition of the emotion of fear is particularly affected. Both the recognition and the expression of an emotion such as fear or disgust can be impaired by localized brain damage. There can be a range of different possible responses to each emotion, such as the initiation of calling versus freezing in young monkeys in a fearful situation. Different emotions, as well as different aspects of the same emotion, appear to be modulated by different brain areas and/or different neurotransmitters.

2.5 Basic emotions: evidence from brain imaging

Brain-imaging procedures offer the opportunity to explore emotion in healthy human volunteers. However, information about brain localization and the distinctiveness of the basic emotions yielded by any one study can be somewhat limited. It is difficult to make sense of it all if different studies indicate that different brain areas are important. A useful technique in these situations, called a meta-analysis, pools the results from many studies to explore which brain areas are most consistently activated for each emotion. Areas of relative regional specialization for fear, anger and disgust have been identified using this method (Murphy *et al.*, 2003). Happiness and sadness were not found to differ significantly from one another in terms of their overall patterns of neural activity, although the patterns of activity do differ from those of the other 'basic' emotions. Figure 2.11 indicates the percentage of studies in which specific brain regions are activated.

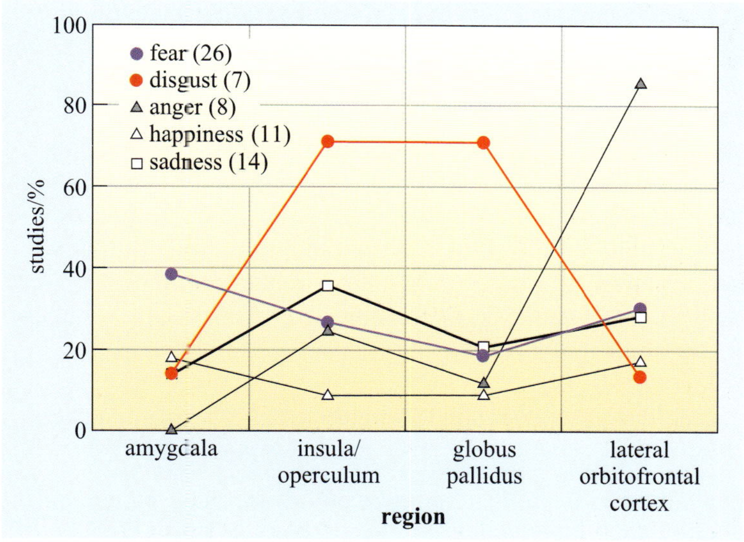

Figure 2.11 The proportion of studies from the meta-analysis targeting the emotions of fear, disgust, anger, happiness and sadness that activated the brain regions associated most consistently with each of those emotions. The number in brackets in the key is the number of studies included in the meta-analysis for that emotion.

- Which emotion is associated with amygdala activation in the highest proportion of studies?

- Fear, as suggested by earlier research, activates the amygdala most reliably in almost 40% of studies.

In contrast to the brain lesion studies reported earlier, the lack of activation in the amygdala for the emotion of anger may seem surprising and, although most often implicated in the fear emotion, slightly over 60% of fear studies do not indicate significant activation in this area. This conflicting evidence reflects some of the limitations of this type of study. In brain-imaging experiments, brain activation in response to a particular emotion must be compared with the activation following neutral or other emotions (Book 3, Section 2.4.1). In order to provide enough data and statistical power, the comparisons, for example between fear and neutral emotions or between neutral and happy emotions, must be repeated a number of times in a single imaging session lasting usually less than one hour. The emotions elicited must necessarily be mild if they are to switch several times in a single session. Additionally, the restrictions of the testing situation, with the participant lying very still and with limited viewing and responding options available, also restrains the intensity of emotion that can be studied. Imaging studies therefore often involve merely viewing pictures of emotion expressions, or viewing pleasant versus unpleasant pictures. Alternatively, participants may be asked to recall past autobiographical episodes during which they felt particular emotions. In Figure 2.11, the 'anger' studies required participants either to identify facial expressions or to recall angry autobiographical situations. These methods limit the intensity and realism of emotion, and therefore the probability of reliably detecting brain activation localized in particular brain regions. They contrast with the more intense emotions often elicited in some lesion studies.

Based on evidence from brain-damaged individuals, a number of emotion researchers have suggested that the right hemisphere of the brain has a more dominant role than the left hemisphere in processing emotions. This hypothesis has also been scrutinized using the above meta-analysis of a large number of brain-imaging studies. It revealed that approximately equal numbers of studies noted maximum activations located in the left and the right hemispheres. A suggested distinction between positive and negative emotions also failed to suggest dominance by either hemisphere. A hemisphere imbalance only arises when considering emotion in terms of its associated motivational tendencies. Emotions can be thought of as leading broadly to the alternative tendencies of approach (e.g. rewards or anger) or withdrawal (e.g. avoidance in fear or disgust). In the overall analysis of imaging studies, this distinction did yield differences between the two hemispheres, with the left being more often or more intensely activated for approach emotions, whilst both were equally activated for withdrawal emotions. Approach motivation can follow from both pleasant and negative emotions, e.g. in anticipating a reward as well as threatening behaviour in anger. Withdrawal motivation arises from fear, but sadness may represent absence of approach tendencies rather than active withdrawal.

- ◆ What other brain function has been found to be very strongly localized in one hemisphere?
- ◆ In Book 5, Section 2.3.2 you learnt that language processing takes place predominantly in one side of the brain, the left hemisphere.

The question of laterality in the processing of emotions is still open to much debate. For the moment, then, the promise that brain-imaging techniques might clarify issues of precise spatial location in emotions has yet to be completely fulfilled. The importance of the involvement of areas such as the amygdala are, however, somewhat supported by imaging studies even though there are inconsistencies. These studies suggest that it might be fruitful to consider the similarities and contrasts between different approach and withdrawal motivation emotions. They further indicate that research focused on basic emotions is likely to yield important data on the neural underpinnings of human emotion.

2.5.1 The amygdala and the pathways of fear

In the search for distinct brain areas that might be associated with the basic emotions, we have not so far paid much attention to how these areas might be linked together to form pathways. Much of what we know about brain pathways in emotion has come from studies of fear and fear conditioning, with other emotions studied rather little. Extensive studies using lesions, electrical recording or stimulation and tracing techniques have yielded evidence of two distinct pathways of fear (LeDoux, 1998), both of which involve the amygdala. These two pathways were introduced in Book 1, Section 4.3.2. The amygdala is so important that it has sometimes been described as the 'sensory gateway to the emotions'.

- From Book 1, can you recall the major distinction between the two pathways?
- ◆ One pathway involves cortical structures and can give rise to conscious perception of fear whilst the alternative, quicker route is subcortical and non-conscious.

- Is the processing of emotions special in having such dual pathways?
- ◆ No. You may recall other examples such as the ventral and dorsal stream in the visual pathway (Book 1, Section 4.4.2; Book 4, Section 2.4).

LeDoux found that although the cortical route was required for learning new fear associations, once learnt, the fear responses would still be displayed even if the cortical areas were later damaged. The cortex was still necessary, however, for making fine discriminations between different features of the situation. For instance, in classical conditioning two tones might be presented in the learning situation, only one of which (the conditioned stimulus) is paired with electric shock (the unconditioned stimulus), while the other is presented alone and not paired with any programmed event. In a normal animal, only the tone paired with the shock produces fear but, with damage to the cortical regions, both tones become equally effective in producing fear.

In parallel experiments using the same classical conditioning method, electrical activity within the amygdala itself has been tracked as learning progressed. Before learning, the amygdala is insensitive to both tones, but after training, electrical responses can be recorded after the animal hears the shock-paired tone but not the benign tone. Behaviour follows the same path, with a fear response emerging to the shock-paired tone but not to the other tone. Subsequent lesions of the amygdala always lead to the abolition of this, and other, fear responses.

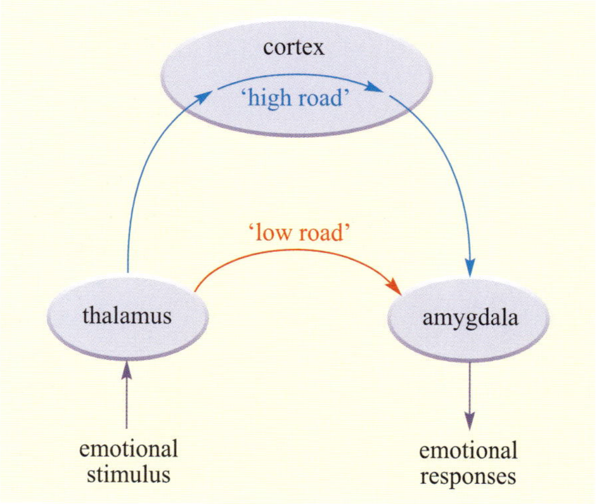

Figure 2.12 Information about external stimuli reaches the amygdala by way of a direct pathway from the thalamus ('low road') as well as by a pathway from the thalamus to the cortex ('high road') to the amygdala. The direct thalamo-amygdala path is shorter and thus a faster transmission route than the pathway from the thalamus through the cortex to the amygdala. However, because the direct pathway bypasses the cortex, it is unable to benefit from cortical processing. As a result, it can only provide the amygdala with a crude representation of the stimulus. It is thus a 'quick and dirty' processing pathway. However, to some extent its utility requires that the cortical pathway is able to override the direct pathway.

Figure 2.12 shows a simplified diagram of the important features of the two pathways that LeDoux has dubbed the 'high road' (slower and passing through the cortex), and the 'low road' (faster but less specific, resulting in 'quick and dirty' processing).

Sensory information from the kinds of stimuli that lead to a fear emotion (such as loud noise, pain, approach of a predator) enters via the thalamus (the part of the thalamus that receives sensory inputs) and then takes two separate routes. The 'low road' is shorter, and thus transmits information more rapidly. It passes directly to the amygdala and thence triggers emotional responses. Since this route bypasses cortical processing, it can respond only to simple biologically threat-relevant stimuli or to relatively crude features of well-learnt, fear-conditioned stimuli. This pathway allows rapid responses to be made to potentially dangerous stimuli, or features of stimuli, before there is time for processing to the point of conscious awareness to be completed. In response to a sudden loud noise or a threatening looming movement, instant freezing or rapid evasive action will be initiated within milliseconds of detection. This can be very useful in dangerous situations. The 'high road', on the other hand, is a longer, slower pathway that passes through cortical regions. To some extent it is capable of overriding the response initiated by the direct pathway and can modify or inhibit other responses according to complex and subtle differences in circumstances through learning. It is possible that the direct pathway is responsible for the control of emotional responses that we do not understand. This may occur in all of us some of the time, but may be a predominant mode of functioning in individuals with certain emotional disorders.

The action of these two routes is readily illustrated with LeDoux's own example (slightly adapted – author's alterations to the quote are in *italics*).

> Imagine walking in the woods. A crackling sound occurs. *The neural signal* generated by the sound goes straight to the amygdala through the thalamic pathway. *The signal* also goes from the thalamus to the cortex. *Cortical processing results in recognition* of the sound as corresponding to either that of a dry twig that snapped under the weight of your boot, or that of a rattlesnake shaking its tail. But by the time the cortex *has registered this (and any additional) ambiguity,* the amygdala is already starting to defend against the snake. The information received *directly* from the thalamus is unfiltered and biased towards evoking responses. The cortex's job is to prevent*/dampen/ reverse* the inappropriate response rather than produce the appropriate one. Alternatively, suppose there is a slender curved shape in the path. *Information regarding the relatively crude features of* curvature and slenderness reach the amygdala from the thalamus, whereas only the cortex distinguishes a coiled up snake from a curved stick. If it is a snake, the amygdala is ahead of the game. From the point of view of survival, it is better to respond to potentially dangerous events as if they were in fact *a threat* than to fail to respond. The cost of treating a stick as a snake is less, in the long run, than the cost of treating a snake as a stick.
>
> (LeDoux, 1998)

Our discussions so far might suggest that the amygdala is one more or less unified structure with only one main type of output (generalized 'emotional responses'). This is something of an over-simplification, its structure is quite complex containing a number of subdivisions or nuclei. In addition, there are numerous output pathways. LeDoux and others have identified that, for fear at least, different pathways from the amygdala are responsible for different types or aspects of the fear response (see Figure 2.13). Earlier in this chapter (especially Section 2.3), we highlighted not only the distinction between different basic emotions, but also the different aspects to emotions (such as recognition/feelings/physiological responses/ expressions) and indeed different responses to the same or similar emotions (such as freezing or calling in fear). When lesion- or brain-imaging studies point towards involvement of the amygdala (as a whole) it may be that function is actually much more focused in different pathways both within it and from it. Just as distinct pathways from the amygdala have been found to be crucial for different aspects of fear, so we might expect that new techniques might further refine the delineation of discrete sub-areas of the amygdala involved with different aspects of other emotions, as well as differentiate between areas involved with the different types of emotion. Further pathways also return to the cortical areas, such as the visual cortex, influencing the processing of signals from sensory inputs.

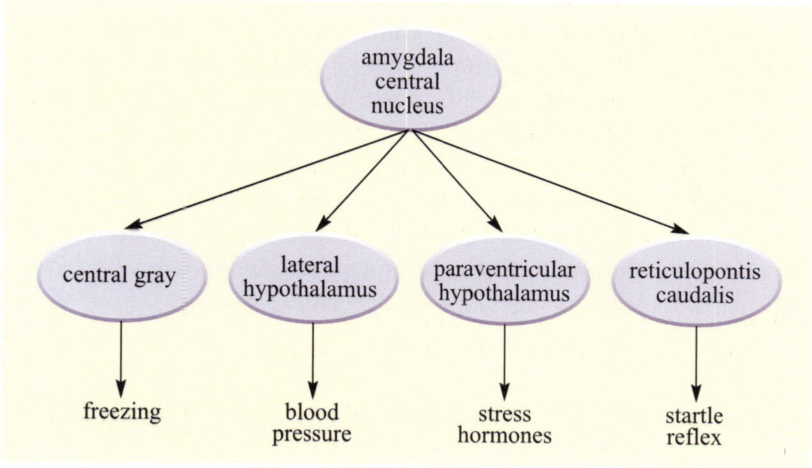

Figure 2.13 Different outputs from the amygdala control different aspects of the fear response. In the presence of danger, or stimuli that might warn of danger, a number of different behavioural and physiological responses are expressed, and the sensitivity to some reflexes, such as the startle reflex, is modulated. Each of these responses is controlled by a different set of outputs from the central nucleus of the amygdala. Damage to the central nucleus blocks the expression of all of these responses, whereas damage to the separate outputs blocks only the individual responses controlled by that pathway. Note: you do not need to recall the names of these different nuclei.

2.5.2 The hippocampus and emotion

In the simple fear-conditioning situation just described, where tones became conditioned stimuli, more is learnt than just the connection between tones and shock. The whole context, and not just the predictive properties of the two tones, becomes part of what is learnt. In such an experiment, the rat becomes conditioned to the whole apparatus as well as to the tones. After learning, as soon as it is returned to the learning situation, the rat will display fear responses such as freezing and/or enhanced startle responses even in the absence of tones or shocks. The whole context, i e. all the background stimuli present, become part of a complex conditioned stimulus. In a more natural example, if a rabbit narrowly escapes an encounter with a fox, it will subsequently be fearful not only of the sight and sound of the fox, but also of the situation where the encounter took place, which it will, if possible, avoid visiting in future.

The hippocampus is one area of the brain that appears to be particularly important in processing context and spatial cues, and damage to this area disrupts context conditioning in animals. After learning simple fear conditioning, rats with damage to the hippocampus no longer show fear when replaced in the conditioning context. However, the tone still arouses characteristic fear responses so the fear conditioning to the tone must have been retained in a normal way.

From human studies, it appears that the hippocampus is not just responsible for learning about the context of an emotional situation but also for being able to bring it explicitly to mind. You will recall the example of H.M. (Book 1, Section 1.1.5; Book 5, Section 1.5.1). H.M. had bilateral damage to his hippocampus that impaired his ability to consciously recall past events, including emotional experiences. When patients with bilateral amygdala damage are compared with those having bilateral hippocampal damage, the dissociation between implicit and explicit learning of fear is neatly illustrated. In a conditioning task in which a skin conductance response

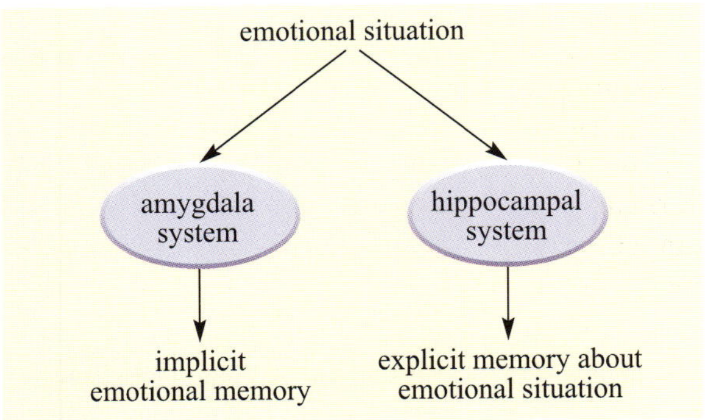

Figure 2.14 Brain systems of implicit and explicit emotional memory.

was measured (see Box 2.3 in Section 2.7), a patient with bilateral amygdala damage was able to report on the conditioning contingencies (e.g. state that a particular tone was followed by a mild shock) but showed no physiological response to the tone: in other words there was no implicit fear conditioning. On the other hand, in a patient with bilateral hippocampal damage but an intact amygdala, the physiological response indicated normal fear conditioning but the patient was unable to recall or report on the learning episode, i.e. there was no explicit knowledge of the conditioning arrangements. Thus, Figure 2.14 illustrates how the inputs from an emotional situation proceed through (at least) two important routes. One route that has already been discussed passes through the amygdala system and gives rise to behavioural and physiological responses to the emotion but without leading to conscious awareness. This route is capable of creating implicit emotional memories and is vital for fear conditioning. The other route, via the hippocampus, is responsible both for context conditioning and for the explicit memories of the emotional situation, i.e. enabling a person to recall the event in the future. If you have been through a traumatic experience and some event triggers your memory later on, you will remember, through the hippocampal system, details of where you were, who you were with, the time of day, and so on. Through the amygdala system, the memory will trigger a rise in heart rate, sweating palms, a churning in the stomach and a sense of unease.

You are not expected to learn or reproduce Figure 2.15, only to notice the complexity of the inputs and outputs involving the amygdala that forms the central hub of the diagram.

What we have described is necessarily a very simplified version of what is known about fear pathways. To give you a flavour of the complexity of possible interactions, Figure 2.15 shows a hypothetical circuit for conditioned fear. This figure is presented only to emphasize the richness of connections and variety of responses involved in just one, apparently simple, emotional pathway.

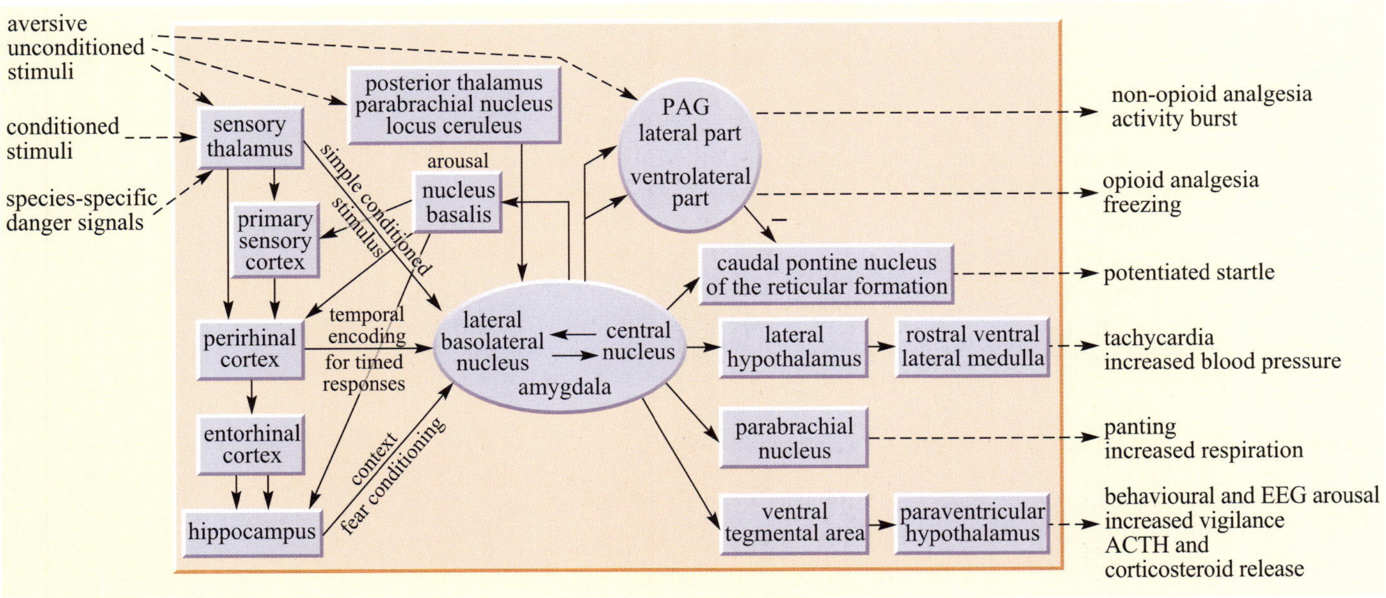

Figure 2.15 Example of a hypothetical circuit showing the different brain areas and pathways thought to be involved in different aspects of the conditioned fear response.

Summary of Section 2.5

During emotional episodes, physiological and behavioural responses are triggered by activity in the limbic system, and the amygdala in particular. A rapid, non-cortical brain pathway from the thalamus directly to the amygdala allows 'quick and dirty' reactions to a potential threat. The amygdala is like the 'hub of a wheel', richly interconnected with other brain areas, for instance it receives low-level inputs from sensory-specific regions of the thalamus, higher-level information from the sensory-specific cortex, and still higher-level (sensory-independent) information about the general situation from the hippocampus. Different aspects of the same emotion are often localized in different regions (nuclei) of the amygdala.

The hippocampus is vital for the conscious explicit recall of emotion memories, but implicit memory is retained if the hippocampus is absent. Different emotions activate some similar and some very distinct regions of the brain. The amygdala seems to be important for all emotions. However, distinct regions or nuclei are often responsible for different emotions as well as different aspects of the same emotion.

2.6 Cognitive models of fear and anxiety

So far, we have tended to consider the processing of fear in a vacuum, without thinking about other features of the situation. In reality, there are nearly always several/many stimuli competing for processing priority. As you will see later (Section 2.9), one function of emotion is to signal the need to interrupt or inhibit current ongoing behaviour to pursue more important goals such as preserving life or seeking pleasure. Interrupting behaviour when danger is imminent makes sense, and this is the type of situation we have considered so far. However, it is also common to encounter signals related to fear/danger that are relatively mild (e.g. a picture of a house on fire or the word 'murder' written in a newspaper). In these cases, urgent action is not required. Indeed, we would rarely get anything done if we responded with a full-blown 'fight or flight' response to every slight suggestion of threat or danger.

Suppose you are giving a brief presentation as part of an important job selection process and there is a commotion outside the room and someone shouts 'fire'. It would probably be wise to stop talking and take action. On the other hand, if those outside the room are just chatting about 'fire', perhaps checking the safety system, then you would rightly ignore their conversation and keep your attention on the task in hand. If you happen to be someone who is particularly anxious about fire, then you might be prone to being particularly easily distracted by hearing its very mention. Your response to whatever matched your current or abiding concern would be amplified in comparison with less-anxious individuals.

Imagine a cognitive psychology experiment in which participants are instructed to respond to a target stimulus in some way, perhaps by pressing one of two buttons as quickly as possible to indicate which of two types of stimulus has been displayed. If a threatening stimulus not relevant to the task is also presented (for a spider phobic an example could be a live spider or a picture of one), then this is likely to attract attention and this distraction could interfere with the speed of responding. Figure 2.16 shows a schematic diagram of how processing of two such potential stimuli might take place. Some preliminary features of the target and the distractor will be rapidly processed and this is represented by the 'target' and 'threat distractor' representation 'boxes' in the figure. (These 'boxes' indicate that some aspects of the input have been registered in the brain (prior to conscious awareness) without suggesting which part(s) of the brain are actually involved.) Before a correct response can be made, attention has to be directed towards the target stimulus so that it can be consciously perceived. The two stimuli will be competing for attention. The relative strength of the output pathway from these 'boxes' determines which stimulus gains attention first, and thus influences the speed of response to the target item. You will notice that the arrows between the target representation and the threat distractor representation have minus signs attached to them. This means that they are mutually inhibitory, in other words as the representation of one increases the more the other is inhibited, and vice versa. A determination to succeed in the task will act to enhance the target representation and thereby suppress that of any distractors. Once the value of a threat distractor becomes sufficiently high, however, its representation begins to inhibit the representation of the target, in turn reducing the target's ability to inhibit the threat, and attention is diverted to threat. The severity of the threat is evaluated by the threat evaluation system. This evaluation is assumed to be influenced by previous learning experiences and modulated by the anxiety levels caused by the person's disposition. For example, a person who has a phobia about spiders might find it particularly hard to ignore the distractor if it was the word tarantula or if the distractor item was a picture of a spider. As an example, the target could be a word and the participant has been asked to indicate as quickly as possible if it is a noun or a verb. The distractor could be another word at a nearby location in the same display. When the distracting threat item is mild (e.g. a word such as hassled), it is easily inhibited (indicated by the minus sign leading from the target representation box to the distractor box) and attention is rapidly directed towards the target in the display. If the threat is more severe, however, (such as the word murder or cancer, or for spider phobics the word spider or tarantula) the activation of the threat distractor representation will be high. In this case, the target representation will be insufficient to inhibit it and attention will become diverted, perhaps only momentarily, towards the threatening item and the task will be disrupted. Anxiety levels, either dispositional or created by past experience or transient mood states, affect how the threat stimulus is evaluated, effectively increasing its 'threat' value and the extent to which it competes for attention. Meanwhile, extra determination to detect and respond to a target in a task helps to inhibit attention to the distracting threat stimulus, but this can only work to a limited degree. It is expected that however hard one tries, sufficiently severe threats will always disrupt the task (and this is the best strategy in the face of real danger, of course). Once attention becomes diverted towards the threat, its threat value is processed more fully. This in turn is likely to increase anxiety further, making it even harder to suppress attention to threats, magnifying interference and disruption to the ongoing task.

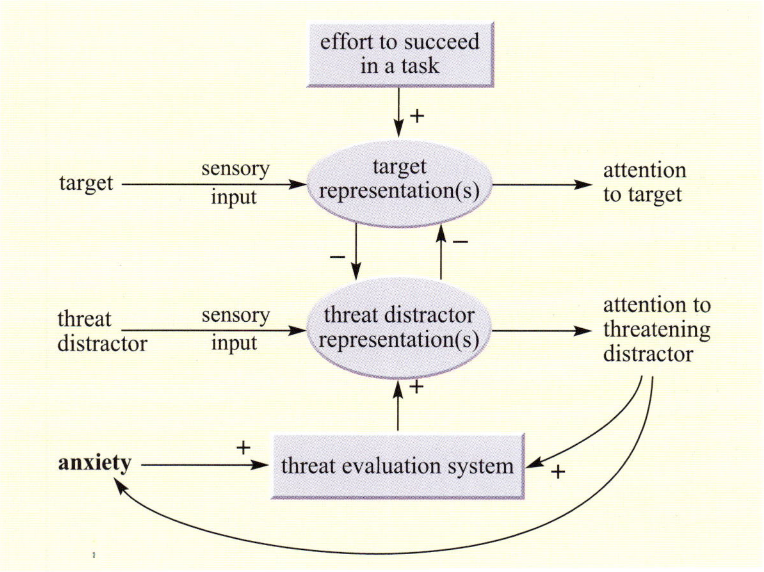

Figure 2.16 A schematic cognitive model of the processing of target and threatening distractor items during a task.

- From the information given earlier in the chapter, which part of the brain seems likely to be involved in the threat evaluation system?

- Although the model does not specify where in the brain different functions take place, the amygdala might be expected to have a role in detecting and evaluating threat.

This type of model helps to contrast the cognitive and the neurobiological approaches to understanding emotions. Whilst neuroscientists such as LeDoux seek to identify neural pathways, cognitive scientists try to make sense of everyday behaviour and performance in cognitive tasks. Integration of these two approaches improves both. For instance, increased knowledge about brain pathways should lead cognitive models to point towards specific brain areas that might serve the various processing stages suggested. Activations can then be mapped using brain imaging whilst participants perform cognitive tasks. Although the 'boxes' in the cognitive model in Figure 2.16 are not (at this stage) intended to map onto specific identifiable brain areas, it is assumed that the threat evaluation system involves the amygdala, including the hippocampus when context is important. Evidence suggests that the amygdala is more readily activated in anxious individuals. Task demand seems to be a frontal lobe activity. (Remember Phineus Gage, Book 1, Section 1.1.4, who became easily distracted and uninhibited in his emotions after damage to his frontal lobes.) The inhibitory links in the model might well be located in the anterior cingulate cortex since this region seems to be activated whenever there is conflict within or beween tasks, or when distracting information must be inhibited.

2.7 Physiological responses and the experience of emotion

When we describe our emotional experiences, we regularly refer to some part of the body or aspect of bodily reaction in the process: a broken/pounding/fluttering heart, butterflies/knot in the stomach, gut feelings, hairs at the back of the neck standing on end, pale/flushed face, and so on. You have already learnt about the coordinated set of responses by the autonomic nervous system (ANS) that are triggered in response to danger (Book 1, Sections 2.3.1 and 3.5.1). Connections between such physiological responses and the experience of emotion form part of a number of sometimes contrasting theories about their roles. Two such theories are explained in Box 2.2. The James–Lange theory assumes that differences in the response to an emotional stimulus/situation provide information for differentiating emotions, i.e. the emotion that you feel is determined by your response. You do not cry because you are sad, nor run away because you are afraid, but feel sad because you cry and feel afraid because you flee. This may seem a rather counterintuitive way for emotions to arise. An alternative notion, such as suggested in the Cannon–Bard theory, reverses the order and suggests that you feel a particular emotion and that in turn initiates the body's reaction.

What evidence is there to support this controversy? In the James–Lange theory, different emotions can only be experienced if different somatic or physiological responses arise in each case. However, when Cannon suggested his theory, it was assumed that visceral responses were the same for all emotions. Since then, evidence has been sought for distinctiveness of physiological responses for each emotion. In an often-quoted study, Ax (1953) measured 14 physiological responses in an elaborate experiment designed to invoke fear and anger. In this experiment, the participants were led to believe that they were taking part in a study on hypertension. They were either confronted with a technician whose apparent incompetence suggested they risked an electric shock from faulty equipment (to elicit fear), or with an abusive person (to elicit anger). Participants confirmed, at the end of the study, that the appropriate emotions had been generated by these manipulations. Ax found that seven of the physiological measures showed differences between the two emotions, for instance the increase in pulse rate and blood pressure was much greater for fear than for anger. Similarly, Funkenstein (1955) showed that the adrenal glands respond to fear by releasing proportionately more adrenalin, but react to anger by secreting more noradrenalin.

Box 2.2 Physiological responses and experience of emotion

James–Lange theory

In 1884, American philosopher William James and, independently, in 1885, Danish psychologist Carl Lange, put forward related theories of emotion now commonly known as the **James–Lange theory**. They proposed that we experience emotion in response to physiological changes in our body and not as a direct result of our cognitive appraisal of the situation. We do not therefore run away from a bear because we are frightened, but rather feel frightened because we are running from a bear – the flight response comes before the feeling of fear in their view.

In James's terms (capital letters as in the original):

> ...the bodily changes follow directly the PERCEPTION of the existing fact, and that our feeling of the same changes as they occur IS the emotion.
>
> (James, 1884, p. 189)

According to James and Lange, the physiological changes are the emotion, and if they are removed the emotion will go with them. You may think this idea is ridiculously backward, as others did at the time of its proposal, and assume that emotion is evoked by the situation and physiological responses follow. Before you reject this theory completely, however, try one of the thought experiments suggested by James. Suppose you are extremely angry with someone. Imagine removing all the physiological accompaniments to the anger – your pounding heart slows, your tense muscles (including clenched fists) relax, your flushed face cools. Without these 'body reactions' it is hard to imagine being as full of rage as you were. Or, consider positive emotions for a change; you are about to go on a date with the person you 'fell in love with' last week. You cannot relax, your hands are sweating, your heart racing, you have a feeling of euphoria and excitement. Now imagine sweeping away all those physiological signs. I bet your 'love' now seems lukewarm in comparison!

Although this aspect of the theory has a ring of truth about it, the situation is obviously more complex, since individuals who have had a spine injury preventing some of these physiological reactions still feel emotion, although sometimes in dampened form. The most basic problem with the James–Lange theory is its failure to specify the mechanism by which bodily changes are initiated by the 'perception of the exciting fact'.

Cannon–Bard theory

In 1927, Cannon proposed a theory, later modified by Bard, that emotions can occur independently of physiological changes outside the brain. Their evidence came from animals and humans who still showed emotional reactions such as anger, fear and pleasure, despite a spinal cord injury that prevents all visceral input travelling to and from the brain. Cannon's work also indicated that emotions were 'experienced' before many parts of the body (such as the smooth muscle) had time to react. In other words, we are capable of feeling emotion before the accompanying bodily changes take place. In addition, there seems no reliable correlation between the experience of emotion and the type of physiological change initiated. For example, fear is accompanied by increased heart rate, increased sweating, inhibited digestion etc., but so is 'being in love', or having a fever. How could feeling fear be a consequence of physiological changes if they do not seem to reliably differentiate between emotions?

More recently, measurement of physiological responses for a wider range of emotions has been attempted, for example participants have been asked to imagine themselves re-enacting past emotional experiences of anger, fear, sadness, happiness, surprise and disgust, as well as by trying to induce real instances of fear, anger and happiness. Some differences in the pattern of physiological responses have been found between the emotions, for instance heart rate increases in response to both fear and anger, but increases in body temperature occur only in anger. In real situations, measures such as skin conductance (Box 2.3; Book 1, Section 4.2.3) and head temperature did distinguish between different emotions, but this was not true of imagined emotions. Overall however, it appears that many measures such as skin conductance and facial temperature do *not* reliably vary with specific emotions. The most reliable difference is in heart rate, but even here five comparisons of happiness and anger revealed differences and five did not. One conclusion is that some of the responses may be due to the general arousing nature of all emotions and as such might be similar in each case. Other responses could be specific to different emotions, but emotion comparisons are hard when it is difficult (or perhaps impossible) to equate intensity of emotion in each case.

Box 2.3 Measuring skin conductance by the galvanic skin response (GSR)

The skin conductance response (SCR), often called the galvanic skin response (GSR), is usually measured by attaching two electrodes onto the surface of the skin on the fingers (Figure 2.17) or sometimes on the palm of the hand. The electrodes measure the skin resistance when a minute current passes between them (the current is so minute that the participant cannot detect it). Skin resistance is altered by the amount of sweat present on the surface layers of the skin – water conducts electrical current rather easily. The 'fight or flight' response includes a change in the amount of sweat released as the body anticipates rigorous physical activity and initiates the cooling process in preparation, but almost any change in the arousal state of the organism results in fluctuations in GSR. The GSR is very sensitive and the recording will show a dramatic increase if the participant becomes fearful. However, many other types of situation will also produce a response when measuring GSR; for instance, general interest in a stimulus, pleasure, laughter, disgust, body movement, and so on. The GSR has been used as a simple 'lie-detector' as the arousal caused by deliberately telling a lie can often be detected, even when the lie results from complying with instructions, such as an experimenter asking a participant to give the wrong answer to half the questions they ask. However, practice can modify the 'lie' response but usually there remains an alternative indicator of effort, such as a change in GSR response in preparation for the question. Deliberate efforts to relax and become calm will usually result in the trace showing GSR to fall steadily. The response can be very sensitive to change, so that even opening the eyes gently after a period of relaxation with them closed will be enough to create an increase in signal.

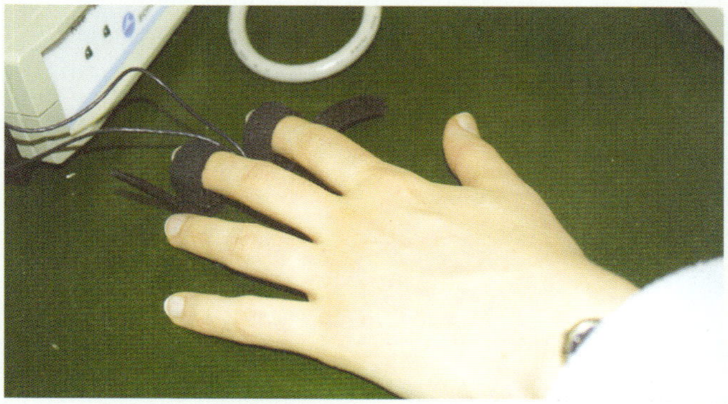

Figure 2.17 Galvanic skin response test.

As the GSR increases in response to many different emotions, it cannot be used to assess which particular emotion is being experienced. GSR appears to measure arousal rather than emotion itself, so it can be used to measure the intensity of an emotional response. Researchers have been able to use it to compare the response to different stimuli, such as how intense the fear response might be to different brief video clips, and it has been a useful tool to explore the role of cognition or appraisal in modifying the response to the same stimulus. In one line of research, participants all watched the same unpleasant film clip. It was a rather gruesome anthropological film showing a rite of passage ritual for adolescent boys. Several alternative sound tracks accompanied the film to help the participants to appraise the film in different ways. The options were:

- no sound track;
- a sound track that emphasized the anthropological interest, that is the script discussed the interesting customs of this native group and pointed out the features of the custom (the intellectualization script);
- a script that denied the pain and trauma experienced by the boys participating and indicated that they were enthusiastic about the experience, which was joyful; they looked forward to this proof of their manhood (the denial script);
- a script which emphasized the trauma being experienced (the trauma script).

The GSR of each participant was recorded while they viewed the film. They all found watching the film moderately distressing, but those who watched it whilst listening to the denial or intellectualization scripts reported less distress when asked afterwards, and this was reflected in an attenuation of the GSR measured whilst they watched.

Figure 2.18 shows a repetition of this experiment, but this time with two different types of denial compared with a silent film. In the *denial commentary*, the sound track emphasized how the boys enjoyed the experience as in the first experiment. However, in the *denial orientation* condition the same information was given in written form before the participants watched the film. The GSR trace for this group shows a marked increase of responding whilst they read the information and try to get ready for the film. After this initial peak, the trace shows that preparing for the film with the denial orientation produces a very marked attenuation of the trace during the film itself, in comparison with the other two groups. These results clearly indicate the importance of appraisal on physiological and self-report measures of arousal and emotion, as well as the importance of preparation to attain an appropriate mindset to avoid distress. Note, in each trace, a period of 'baseline' measurements assess the pre-film levels of GSR for comparison with the 'during film' trace.

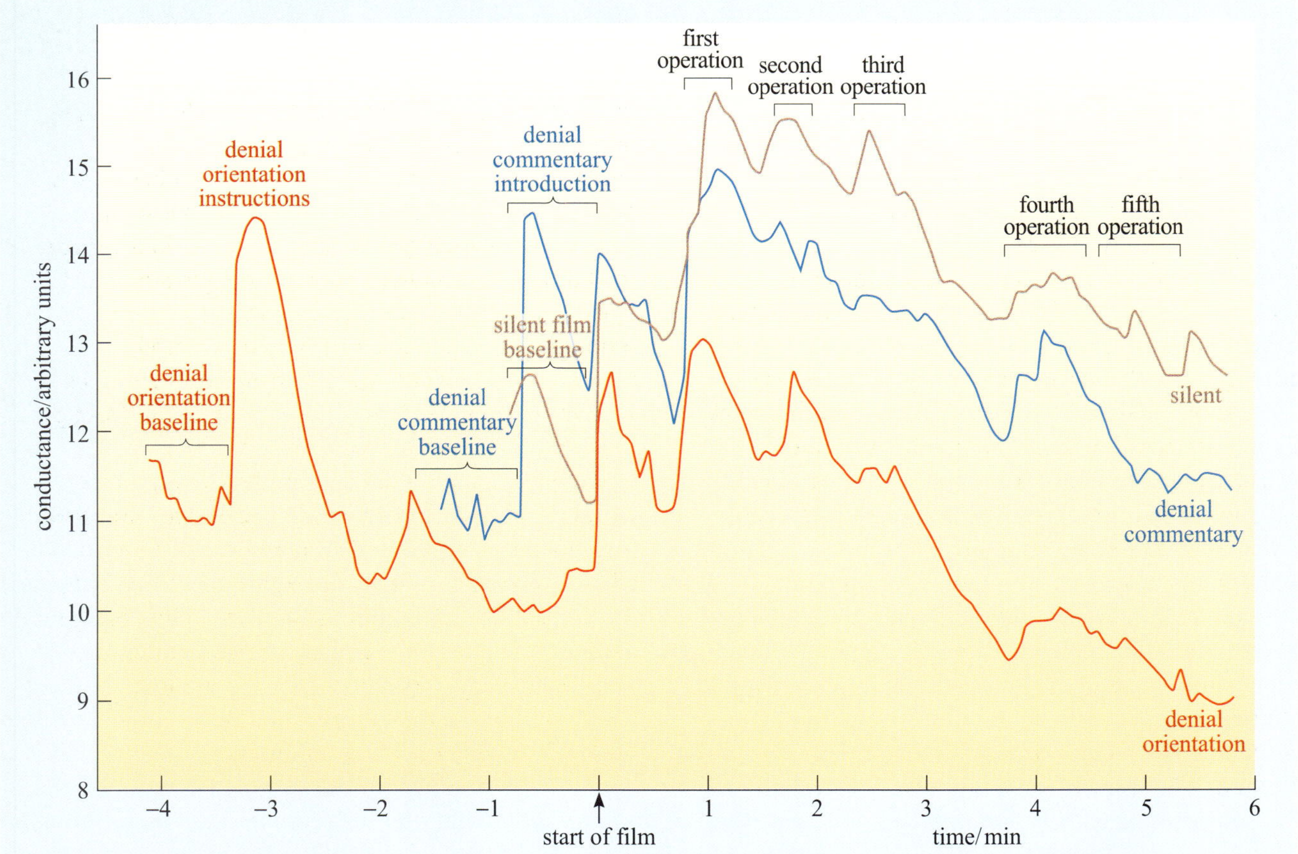

Figure 2.18 Skin conductance responses taken before and during the period when different groups of participants watched a film involving adolescent boys receiving unpleasant rite of passage operations.

It is probably the case that not all emotions are associated with exactly the same type of autonomic response, although there may well be some shared features. Does this offer support for the James–Lange theory? Regardless of whether they are sufficiently differentiated, the visceral responses are mostly too slow (taking sometimes several seconds to arise) and long-lived to determine the emotion felt at any particular moment. Emotions may fluctuate rapidly over time, such as when fear gives way to anger then humour during a practical joke, and happiness turns to despair as you watch your team-mate trip and fall moments short of winning an important race.

- If the James–Lange theory were correct, what should happen to the emotional experience of someone suffering from spinal injury that prevented many or all visceral responses?

- The prediction would be that they would not be able to feel emotion nor distinguish between different emotions. Although such individuals may sometimes suffer from blunted reactions, their emotional experiences are not destroyed by the injury.

Does this suggest acceptance of the Cannon–Bard account? Before you answer, have a look at Box 2.4 on how physiological responses may influence emotional experience, and you will see that both theories have some support.

Box 2.4 Influence of physiological responses on emotional experience

Two researchers, Schachter and Singer, argued that both cognitive and physiological aspects of emotion are important and that when either component is missing, the emotional experience is incomplete. In their original study (1962), they investigated the effects of participants' reactions to an injection of adrenalin. Some participants were told of the actual effects of the drug (increased heart rate, shaking and flushing of the face), others were given incorrect information, and others were given no information at all. Schachter and Singer manipulated the kind of experience that followed the injection by introducing a fellow worker (confederate) to the group. Some participants waited with a confederate who behaved in a happy playful manner, others with a confederate who was angry and aggressive. On the basis of observed behaviour and self-reports, those participants who did not attribute the physiological reactions to the drug were greatly influenced by the confederate, becoming more happy or angry in comparison to the correctly informed participants.

In another study, Dutton and Aron (1974) contrived to manipulate participants' feelings about an attractive confederate that they met on either a high or a low bridge. The assumption was that whilst walking across a high and slightly precarious bridge the body would produce some of the physiological reactions appropriate to fear. If, whilst in the process, you meet someone whom you find attractive, the pounding heart (from fear) could be incorrectly appraised as a racing heart from 'falling in love'. This is exactly the result that the researchers found. The same confederate met participants on either a high or low bridge and asked them to complete a questionnaire, leaving a telephone number to allow participants to follow up the contact later. When compared with 'low bridge' participants, more of the 'high bridge' participants made follow-up contacts, which the authors interpreted as a differential attraction for the confederate, fuelled by the adrenalin.

As is often the case, there seem to be elements of truth in both ideas, i.e. the James–Lange theory and the Cannon–Bard theory. How can this be resolved? The clue might be provided by the observation that emotions are very dynamic. The James–Lange theory might well be correct as a description of the first response to an emotional situation. In Book 1, Section 4.3.2, and Section 2.5.1 of this chapter, you came across the 'quick and dirty' brain pathway involved in fear that allows rapid responses to be made even before we have time to be consciously aware of the danger. The theory is correct in assuming that the defensive fear reaction precedes the feeling of fear. Next, the slower cortical appraisal of the situation is able to modify the emotional equation, if necessary. But feelings are by no means static. The current external stimuli (which could be being rapidly updated, e.g. if you were fleeing), as well as stimulation provided by your body movements and physiological reactions, all provide further sensory input. Along with current cognitive appraisals, this information becomes part of a feedback loop that is again processed by the slow and fast, conscious and non-conscious mechanisms. These recompute the current emotional status at each cycle, based on the additional and updated information now available (including the perception of individuals of their ability to cope with the situation, and their actual coping responses), as the emotional experience unfolds (Figure 2.19).

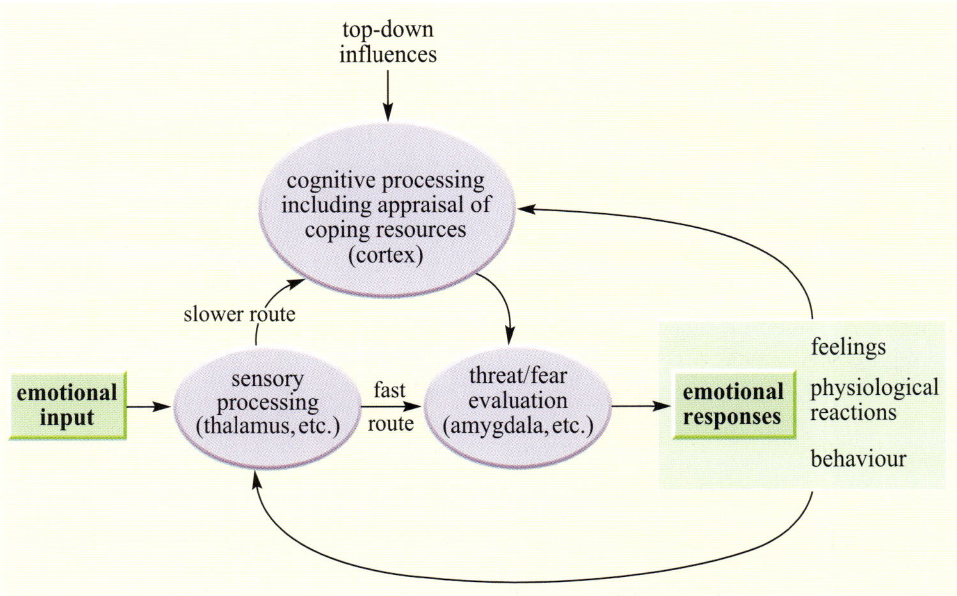

Figure 2.19 Schematic diagram of possible cycles of feedback and cognitive appraisal as an emotional response develops.

There are many features that could be added to this figure since emotional responses and experience are modulated further by a range of factors, such as individual differences in temperament, competing processing, attentional set (what is being attended to), and so on. Figure 2.20 illustrates how the magnitude of the simple startle reflex can be exaggerated (potentiated) by the presence of a fear stimulus or unpleasant picture, or reduced if a person is viewing something else that is interesting or pleasant. In animals, the startle reflex is enhanced when the animal is exposed to a signal that has previously signalled unpleasant events such as shock. In humans, the startle is reduced if a sudden sound occurs whilst they are looking at something interesting and/or pleasant or, alternatively, it is exaggerated if they are viewing something unpleasant. These examples are important because the startle reflex is very fast, and is organized at brainstem level. There is no time for it to be influenced by passing through the slow cortical route. As the brain processes events to evaluate their emotional content, for instance using pathways leading from the cortex to the amygdala, there are also pathways leading back from the amygdala towards the cortex that will modify further inputs. In this way, inputs leading from the amygdala can serve to modulate the extent of the startle response – the amygdala is richly interconnected with many other brain areas so we must bear in mind how complex the emotion pathways are in their detail.

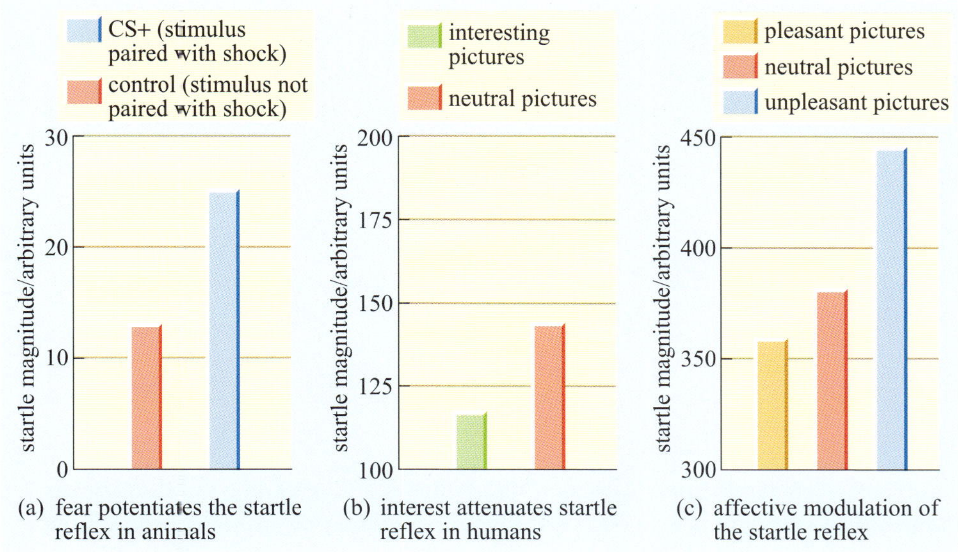

Figure 2.20 Potentiated startle responses. (a) Startle reflexes are potentiated in animals when a cue signals shock, compared with a no-shock condition (control); (b) startle reflexes are inhibited when human subjects look at interesting compared with neutral pictures; (c) startle reflexes are potentiated when viewing unpleasant pictures as well as inhibited when viewing pleasant pictures, compared with neutral pictures, producing affective modulation of the startle reflex.

- From the data in Figure 2.20, when is the startle response greatest?
- The startle response is greatest in the presence of an unpleasant stimulus, either an unpleasant picture (for humans) or a conditioned stimulus (CS) that has been paired with shock (for animals). The exaggerated response in the presence of the conditioned stimulus that has been paired with shock is an example of fear-potentiated startle.

In Box 2.5, you will see there is some evidence for feedback from facial expressions to emotional experience. Our consideration of the importance of feedback from physiological responses to the cortex (Figure 2.19) would be incomplete if we failed to make reference to the ideas of Antonio Damasio. He suggests that physiological reactions to emotional situations form part of the richness that makes up each emotional experience, but that we also use feedback from the physiological reactions to help in decision making as so-called 'somatic markers'. His idea is that when we come to situations where we need to make a

Box 2.5 Do you smile because you are happy or are you happy because you smile?

You may think it is silly to suppose that just putting a smile on your face is what makes you happy, but there is certainly evidence that facial expressions influence how you feel.

Ask someone to hold a pen between their teeth without touching it with their lips, partially mimicking a smile. They will be more likely to judge a cartoon as being funnier compared with another person holding a pen firmly between their lips without touching it with their teeth (simulating a frown), or report feeling happier when watching neutral and emotionally charged slides (Figure 2.21).

Of course, if you would really like to try this out, you will have learnt by now that you will need a fair number of people doing each task, as well as an appropriate control group!

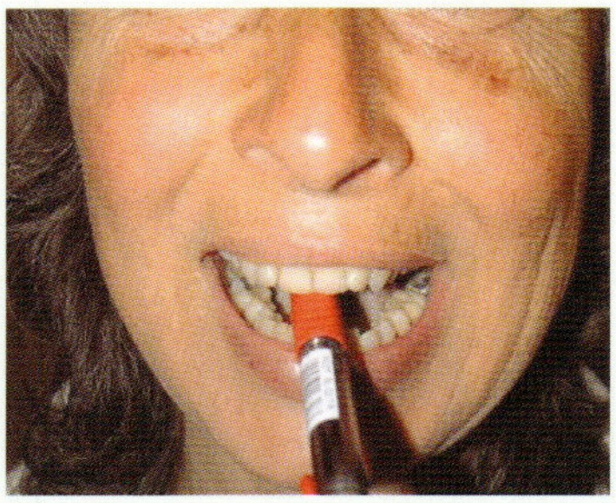

(a)

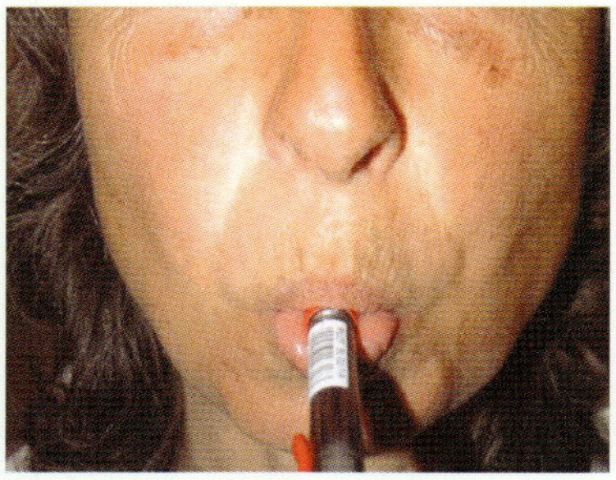

(b)

Figure 2.21 A technique to induce subjects to (a) smile or (b) not smile without their awareness.

choice between several possibilities we may imagine making one or other choice in turn. If the thought of one choice leads to a particular physiological sensation, sometimes informally called a 'gut reaction', then we can use that information to assist us in making the decision about which option to select. Research on this topic has centred on a task in which participants turn over cards from four possible decks of cards. Cards in two of the decks lead on to small rewards and small fines, resulting in a small gain over time. Cards in the other two decks lead to occasional large rewards but also to large punishing fines so that on average a loss is made if selections are made from these packs. Over time, most normal participants settle for making choices from the two small-reward 'safe' decks. Damasio suggests that, as we repeat experiences of reward and punishment, distinct physiological responses become conditioned to the two types of deck. When we contemplate picking cards from each deck this response becomes a 'somatic marker' that can guide our choice without the need for any explicit or conscious knowledge of why the choice was made. This leads to the prediction that any individual who cannot generate the appropriate physiological response will perform poorly at this task. This prediction is upheld for some patients with brain damage, particularly in the amygdala. This can lead to overly risky decisions and socially inappropriate behaviour in their everyday lives as they are unable to use gut reactions to guide decision making or anticipate the outcome of their interactions with others.

2.8 Previous experience

2.8.1 Early experience

In Book 3, Section 3.4.1 you learnt how, in rats, experience during rearing affects later behaviour in an Open Field. The Open Field Test provides a measure of fearfulness: fearful animals avoid the exposed central area of the test arena. Rat mothers that provide high levels of grooming and licking reared less-fearful youngsters. Gray (1987) reports how even prenatal events (stressing the mothers) could influence sensitivity to fearful situations. In another careful cross-fostering study, rats whose mothers had been exposed to severe stress before their birth were more fearful later.

- Why was it important to cross-foster the infant rats?
- Although the mother rats were no longer stressed after their infants were born, prior stress could have altered their rearing behaviour. To be sure that it was the prenatal experience, rather than the influence of the mother, cross-fostering is essential. Look back to Book 3, Section 3.4 for a discussion about controlling these types of confounding variables.

In another series of experiments, Gray reports how an additional aspect of early treatment in rats modulates responses to fear later on. In this research, early handling by experimenters, or other mild stresses, reduced fear reactions later in what is often described as a kind of 'emotional immunization' or 'stress inoculation'. You will see later how genetic factors also play a part in the fear response of rats Many studies suggest that, just as for rats, the complex interactions between early experience and genes influence individual differences in reactivity to fear in humans, and similar effects are likely to be true of other emotions. In Book 3, Section 3.9.2, you have already seen an example of the way aggressive behaviour in humans can arise through an interaction between genes and childhood experiences.

2.8.2 Learning and memory

- In descriptions of conditioning studies such as those in Book 5, Section 1.2, what features do the unconditioned stimuli, reinforcers or punishers have in common?
- They are all stimuli that evoke an emotional response. By pairing a previously neutral stimulus with an emotionally charged one, the neutral stimulus becomes emotionalized, e.g. a tone that has been paired with shock elicits fear after conditioning whereas previously it was neutral.

In the conditioning studies, we emphasized how learning about connections between previously neutral stimuli and emotional events (unconditioned stimuli) takes place so that the neutral stimuli become emotionalized themselves. The mere presence of emotionally arousing stimuli can influence other aspects of memory such that moderate stress occurring during memory consolidation enhances memory, although explicit memory might be impaired if the stress is too severe. As we have seen already, emotional stimuli activate the amygdala and hippocampus. Imaging studies with humans support the conclusions reached in earlier work on animals suggesting that the amygdala and hippocampus play a crucial role in the modulation of memory function. In the example in Figure 2.22, positive correlations between glucose uptake in both these structures and later recall of pleasant but not neutral pictures are shown (see Book 2, Section 1.2.6 for a discussion about correlations).

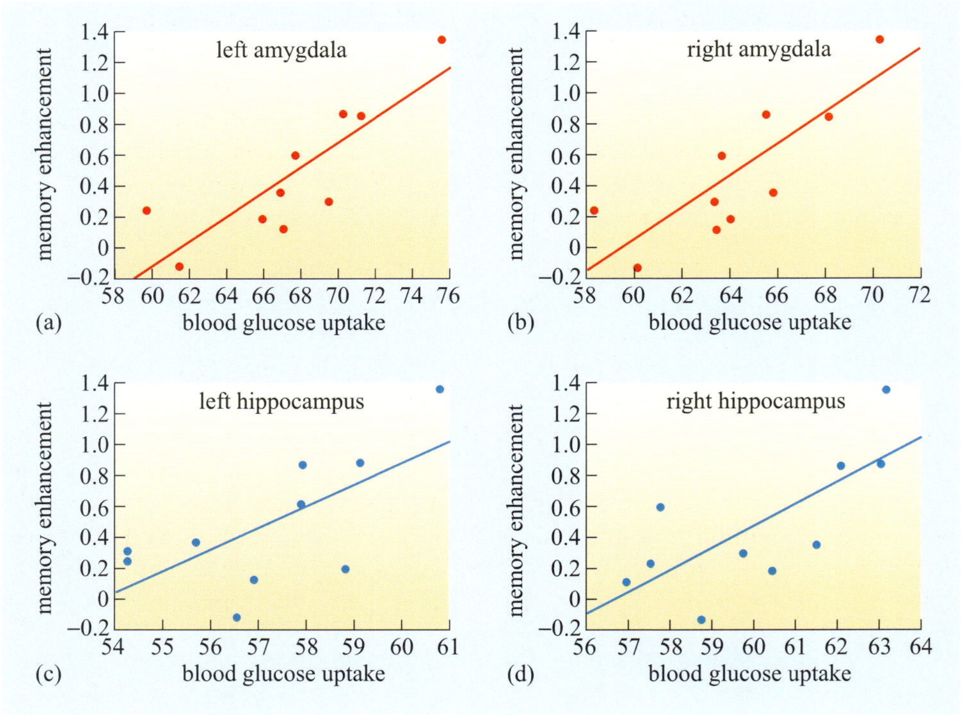

Figure 2.22 The relationship between pleasant-picture memory and brain activity for ten participants. Memory enhancement is defined as recognition for pleasant pictures minus recognition for neutral pictures (the amount by which memory for pleasant pictures exceeds that for neutral pictures), and is indicated on the vertical axis of the graph with larger (positive) numbers indicating relatively more accurate recognition in comparison with neutral pictures. The measurement of blood glucose uptake in the brain areas considered is shown on the horizontal axis. Higher numbers along the horizontal axis indicate higher levels of blood glucose uptake. (a) and (b) Correlation plots for the left and right amygdala; (c) and (d) correlation plots for the left and right hippocampus.

- ◆ From Figure 2.22, describe the relationship between amygdala and hippocampal activity and the recognition of pictures.

- ◆ In the figure there is a positive correlation between both hippocampal and amygdala activity and recall (recognition enhancement). In other words, better memory was shown for those stimuli (the more emotional ones) that activated the hippocampus and amygdala the most, causing enhanced uptake of blood glucose. (Remember that an increased uptake of blood glucose in a particular brain area indicates increased activity in that area.)

  Similar results were also found for films with a frightening content, which therefore enhanced memory through negative emotions.

Book 1, Section 4.3 highlighted the existence of non-conscious processing of events. Very simple learning can take place with stimuli that do not reach consciousness, and that section described how subliminal presentations of happy and fearful faces activated the amygdala despite the fact that only the interleaved neutral faces reached awareness. In similar experiments, the neutral faces were rated to indicate how pleasant/unpleasant they seemed after being paired with happy and fearful faces. Those paired with happy faces were liked more than those paired with fearful faces.

In Book 1, Sections 1.1.6 and 4.3.2, we discussed the notion of subliminal stimuli (i.e. stimuli presented too briefly to reach awareness) and even the possibility that they might influence learning. What happens when such subliminal stimuli are repeated often? Does 'familiarity breed contempt'? In what is known as the 'mere exposure effect', pre-exposed stimuli are generally rated as more pleasant than equivalent novel ones even when they have been exposed subliminally, so that viewers are completely unaware that they have seen them before.

Along with what you already know about learning and memory, these few examples illustrate the considerable opportunities for stimuli in our environment to become emotionalized. It may also help you to understand the psychology behind some advertising campaigns: present your new, initially neutral, product many times, preferably alongside something your target audience finds pleasant and attractive; repeat this sequence enough times and the neutral product will acquire emotional qualities of its own – it will be rated as more desirable or pleasant. It does not matter, of course, whether the 'pleasant' item for pairing has anything whatever to do with the product. A beautiful/handsome model draped over a new car is a good example. However, don't worry too much about being inadvertently 'brainwashed' by so-called subliminal advertising. Subliminal effects are usually very mild and require lots of repetitions.

Summary of Section 2.8

There are a number of ways that previously neutral stimuli can be paired with emotional stimuli and become emotionalized. Simply becoming familiar with neutral stimuli is likely to make them appear more pleasant. Emotional arousal and activation of the amygdala and hippocampus enhance learning.

2.9 Functions of emotion

In Section 2.3.1, we discussed how emotional reactions and displays, especially in Western cultures, are often criticized, and individuals are encouraged to be rational and considered in their decisions. Darwin felt that emotions were a vestige left over from our animal ancestors. Does this mean that emotions do not serve modern humans with any useful function(s)?

- ◆ What is meant by a functional explanation of emotions?
- ◆ Think (or look) back to Book 1, Section 1.4 in which we considered different types of perspective and explanation that might be sought in biological psychology. When we ask questions about the function of emotion we want to consider what advantage if any it might confer in evolutionary terms.

It is easy to find examples where 'following one's emotions' may lead to disaster. As an example, a woman whose bag is stolen by a gang of youths may be better off letting them go than fighting for its retrieval. We shall leave aside the delicate issue of 'falling in love' (mischievously defined by the late Stuart Sutherland in his dictionary of psychology as a form of temporary mental disorder), but are there reasons to be thankful for our emotions?

The short answer is yes. Not all occurrences of emotions necessarily serve a useful purpose, but most biologists and psychologists would agree that on balance they have an adaptive function. The easiest emotion to appreciate is probably fear. In Book 1, Section 3.5.1, you learnt how the body responds with a complex set of physiological reactions to potential or actual threat, putting it into a state of readiness for physical activity, be it flight or fight. This response is initiated very rapidly (remember the 'quick and dirty' pathway of fear), for instance if you are startled by a sudden loud noise you will jump within 20 ms (milliseconds) of its onset (the startle response). You will also rapidly orient towards the source of this stimulus giving it, and your escape route, your full attention. Meanwhile, the other physiological responses to danger, such as increased heart rate, altered blood flow and so on, will already be initiated, boosting blood flow to fuel muscles vital for flight. It will, by most estimations, be at least a further 200 ms before you have had time to become consciously aware of the source and nature of the stimulus and somewhat longer before you make a rational decision about a sensible response to this situation. Your rapid emotional response would have already instigated avoiding action well before the rational decision, let alone response, could be mustered. This time saved could be the difference between life and death. Anger is similar, except that it can prepare for fight rather than flight, providing the rapid physiological resources and boldness to risk a challenge that might be required to protect your own or your loved ones' safety or status.

Likewise, the utility of surprise and disgust may seem fairly easy to guess. The emotion of surprise alerts us to the presence of something novel (or indeed the novel absence of something expected – such as the cessation of the ticking of a clock). When the unexpected occurs, part of the surprise reaction directs attention to assess its significance. Disgust helps to reduce the risk of illness by avoiding contact with potentially dirty or fouled surfaces or refusing the ingestion of foods that might be contaminated, rotting or poisonous.

There is not the space in this book to consider each emotion in turn, but you may be able to think of some useful functions of emotions yourself. Some emotions seem to be more concerned with fulfilling basic needs – think back to Chapter 1 – whilst others such as shame, guilt or humour are associated more closely with building and maintaining social cohesion. But what then is the function of the feelings of these emotions and, for instance, why is there a long period of distress during the process of mourning the death of a loved one?

Emotion researchers such as Oatley and Johnson-Laird (1987) have tried to make sense of this aspect of the function of emotions. In their thinking, based on earlier ideas by Simon (1967), one important role of emotion may be to signal to the organism that ongoing behaviour should be interrupted to take account of a conflicting goal. Humans have many different motivations and goals. Events will happen that require setting or resetting of the priorities amongst these goals, such as giving up the goal of planting next summer's food crop in favour of running away from an attacking lion. Sadness during bereavement, in their framework, is not just a maladaptive waste of time, but can be seen as having the function of initiating readjustment of the life goals that included the lost one. If the association was a close one, this period of reassessing or reforming goals could be lengthy. Table 2.1 summarizes and simplifies some emotions and their proposed functions. The table lists some emotions, suggests an example of the type of event that might elicit the emotion, and the action that might follow from experiencing that emotion. For Oatley and Johnson-Laird, the primary function of the basic emotional signals is related to actions such as increasing, reducing or redirecting how we respond.

Table 2.1 Basic emotions with the functions they perform and the actions that might therefore be accomplished. Emotions in the first group can occasionally be free-floating, i.e. they can occur without the experiencer knowing what caused them; those in the second group always have an object. In this analysis, plans are goal-directed sequences of action.

Emotion (mode)	Eliciting event or object of emotion	Actions
Emotions that can occasionally be free-floating:		
happiness	subgoals being achieved	continue with plan, modifying if necessary; cooperate; show affection
sadness	failure of major plan or loss of active goal	do nothing; search for new plan; seek help
anger	active plan frustrated	try harder; aggress
fear	self-preservation goal threatened or goal conflict	stop current plan; attend vigilantly to environment; freeze and/or escape
Emotions that always have an object:		
attachment love	caregiver	keep contact; talk
caregiving love	offspring	nurture; help; support
sexual love	sexual partner	engage in courtship; sexual activity
disgust	contamination	reject substance; withdraw
contempt	outgroup person	treat without consideration

Happiness might be felt when a goal is progressing well, although we are often too absorbed to notice at the time: it is most likely to be experienced when our goal has finally been successfully achieved. For negative events, interruptions of ongoing behaviour occur after which distinct behaviour patterns are likely to be initiated for different emotions of sadness, anger, fear, and so on. Emotions in the table are divided into those that can be experienced without necessarily knowing what caused them, and those that are always directed towards an object or person. This distinction is also important in determining the action that emerges from the emotion and how it is directed. Thus, emotions function to manage our multiple motives, switching attention from one concern to another when unforeseen events affecting these concerns occur in the world, in the body or in the mind.

Oatley and Jenkins (1996) suggest that it is useful to think of emotional reactions as an inference or best guess providing a rough and ready shortcut for creating prompt action. Even the cleverest of us, provided with unlimited library and computer facilities, would be unable to have access to all the information *in time* to make a rational decision in most situations that give rise to emotions. Moreover, there are often a number of incompatible goals, and no course of action could satisfy them all. The emotional heuristic provides a method of doing something that is usually (but not invariably) useful when there is no guaranteed solution.

In an important paper that influenced Oatley and Johnson-Laird's thinking, Simon (1967) argued that emotions, or their equivalent, are essential for any intelligent being including, if we were able to make it, an intelligent computer. If an intelligent system has a number of different motivations or goals, then something like emotions would be required to set priorities among them, and to allow events to interrupt what the program/individual was doing.

- If emotional expressions do not influence the achievement of our goals, do they have any function, for instance, with respect to other people?

- Expressions transmit information to others about our emotional state. As we are highly social animals this information is immensely useful, such as in indicating to others our intentions. Our expressions on approach to an individual or group may indicate whether we wish to be friendly, submissive or aggressive in our interaction. In turn, we can use the expressions of others to estimate how welcome we are when joining a group, or whether retaliation or fear is the reaction to our aggression.

The scope of this section is too limited to explore many aspects of the functions of emotions but it gives a flavour of some of the issues. Before we leave this topic, however, let us think back to the example of the Capgras' patient introduced in Book 4, Section 2.2. Here the patient recognizes a familiar face, such as his father, yet does not believe it is actually his father because the emotional response is absent. This syndrome illustrates dramatically how unexpectedly vital the role of emotions can be. Visual recognition of a familiar face is not enough. To 'know' it is your father requires activating the emotional response that goes along with everything your father means to you emotionally. Without emotion he is taken for an impostor.

2.10 Emotional disorders

Disorders of mood and emotion, the affective disorders, are not just a problem because of the unhappiness and distress that they bring to us as individuals, but also because of the impact they have on society. They are so common that the World Health Organisation's survey concluded that in 1990 more life-years in midlife were lost to death or disability through clinical levels of depression than through any other source of physical or mental disease or accident (Table 2.2). Rates have risen sharply in the last 50 years and continue to do so.

Table 2.2 The ten leading causes of disease burden in midlife (ages 15–44) throughout the world according to the World Health Organisation, 1996.

Problem	Global cost*
unipolar depression (depression without mania)	42 972
tuberculosis	19 673
road traffic accidents	19 625
alcohol use	14 848
self-inflicted injuries	14 645
bipolar disorder (depression with mania)	13 189
war	13 134
violence	12 955
schizophrenia	12 542
iron-deficiency anaemia	12 511

*The cost is estimated in terms of the number of healthy life-years lost to death or disability as a result of the problem. (As the table considers only mid-life, 15–44 years, this calculation assumes that the average lifespan should exceed 44 years in the absence of disease or accident.)

We all have moments of sadness and gloom, worrying about events that turned out badly, sleeping poorly and lacking motivation to move forwards. We often say we are feeling 'really depressed'.

Likewise, we have all been nervous or anxious about an upcoming event, feeling jittery and restless, unable to relax or sleep soundly.

Conversely, we saw earlier that emotions, even negative ones, can serve a useful function. Does this mean depression and excessive anxiety could even be beneficial?

The answer to these questions is 'probably not' once they interfere with our normal routine (i.e. disrupting sleep patterns), but the fine distinction between what is normal (even helpful) and disordered requiring medical help is often not obvious. Doctors have guidelines to help them make decisions about these disorders. In general, symptoms must persist for several weeks at minimum to be considered abnormal. The most widely used diagnostic criteria are provided by the American Psychiatric Association (Box 2.6).

Box 2.6 Diagnostic criteria for emotional disorders

Doctors use standardized guidelines to diagnose emotional disorders, the most widely used are provided by the American Psychiatric Association. Below are extracts from the 'Diagnostic criteria for depression and generalized anxiety disorder'. To meet the criteria for these conditions, a person must experience the symptoms over an extended period of time.

Diagnostic criteria for depression

The American Psychiatric Association suggest a diagnosis of depression if a person experiences either or both of these primary symptoms:

- persistent feelings of sadness or anxiety;
- loss of interest or pleasure in usual activities;

in *addition* to five or more of these secondary symptoms for at least two consecutive weeks:

- changes in appetite that result in weight losses or gains not related to dieting;
- insomnia or oversleeping;
- loss of energy or increased fatigue;
- restlessness or irritability;
- feelings of worthlessness or inappropriate guilt;
- difficulty thinking, concentrating or making decisions;
- thoughts of death or suicide or attempts at suicide.

Diagnostic criteria for generalized anxiety disorder

Excessive anxiety and worry (apprehensive expectation), occurring more days than not for at least six months, about a number of events or activities (such as work or school performance).

The person finds it difficult to control the worry.

The anxiety and worry are associated with three or (more) of the following six symptoms, with at least some symptoms present for more days than not for the past six months:

- restlessness or feeling keyed up or on edge;
- being easily fatigued;
- difficulty concentrating or mind going blank;
- irritability;
- muscle tension;
- sleep disturbance (difficulty falling or staying asleep, or restless unsatisfying sleep).

The anxiety, worry or physical symptoms cause clinically significant distress or impairment in social, occupational or other important areas of functioning.

The disturbance is not due to the direct physiological effects of a substance (e.g. a drug of abuse, a medication) or a general medical condition (e.g. hyperthyroidism) and does not occur exclusively during a mood disorder, a psychotic disorder or a pervasive developmental disorder.

In generalized anxiety disorder, the focus of anxiety and worry is not confined to those detailed under the criteria for specific anxiety-related disorders. Examples of the symptoms specific to one of the anxiety-related disorders are: worry about having a panic attack (specific to panic disorder), being embarrassed in public (social phobia), being contaminated (obsessive–compulsive disorder), being away from home or close relatives (separation disorder), excessive anxiety about, and attempt to control, body fat despite below average weight (anorexia nervosa), anxiety about having multiple physical complaints (somatization disorder), anxiety about having a serious illness (hypochondriasis), and the anxiety and worry that arise after experiencing a traumatic event (post-traumatic stress disorder). (Note: in other words, all these listed anxiety-related disorders have their own specific diagnoses, which are separately listed in the diagnostic manual. A patient with anxiety problems may meet the criteria for one or more of these other specific disorders, but if their anxiety symptoms do not adequately fit any of these diagnoses but do fulfil the other requirements listed for generalized anxiety disorder then that will be their diagnosis.)

Of the disorders of negative emotions, depression (excessive sadness) and anxiety (excessive fear) seem the most prevalent, and we will touch on them in this chapter. However, we do not have the space to dwell on other disorders. Excessive anger may be more often treated with a prison sentence rather than therapy and excessive disgust or concern with contamination (such as in persistent hand washing) forms one component of the very widespread but largely hidden problem of obsessive–compulsive disorder.

Perhaps it is hard to consider being concerned about excessive happiness, but disorders of positive emotions such as mania may actually constitute a very dangerous state. Mania is accompanied by a state of pathologically high mood. The person feels euphoric and excited, needs little sleep, and is full of new ideas and plans, often for financial gambles or sexual liaisons. His/her thoughts seem to race, and fly from new idea to new idea. This becomes a problem because the person is often so distracted and 'high' that nothing sensible is achieved, which may be as well as ideas may be wildly strange and inadvisable. They can often include hallucinations and grandiose delusions, such as being God or having a special mission. A particular danger is that the euphoria becomes associated with sudden irritability or rage when the rest of the world does not see things the person's way. This can lead to arguments, to violence, and most of all to sudden suicide attempts. Those individuals almost always have episodes of depression as well, and so their condition is called **bipolar disorder** (depression without mania is called **unipolar disorder**). There are reasons for thinking of the bipolar form of the illness as particularly serious, not just because both extremes of mood occur, but also because bipolar sufferers usually have their first episode relatively early in life, with high rates of episode recurrence.

Unipolar and bipolar disorders do not exhaust the spectrum of depressive disorders let alone affective disorders. Depression elicited under particular circumstances attracts special designations, such as seasonal affective disorder (SAD), which is associated with the changing seasons, and post-natal depression, which is associated with childbirth in women. From genetic studies and from the spread of disorders responsive to the same drug treatments, there are reasons for thinking that many disorders such as anxiety, panic attacks, social phobia, eating disorders and obsessive–compulsive disorder are biological relatives, thus they constitute an affective disorder spectrum.

◆ Turn back to Table 2.2. How many of the top ten causes of disability listed might involve the affective disorder spectrum?

◆ As well as unipolar and bipolar disorders, excessive alcohol use and self-inflicted injuries could also denote affective disorder. In addition, some interpersonal violence could also stem from affective problems. If correct, then affective disorders account for an overwhelming majority of midlife disability throughout the world.

2.11 The brain level

Throughout this course we have concentrated on relationships between brain function and behaviour, between biology and psychology. Using depression and anxiety as examples, how might changes in brain function be linked to emotional disorder? Depression involves an attenuation of the normal positive emotional responses, and a pathological increase in the negative ones. We might suspect that this would show up in an altered activity in those parts of the brain thought to be involved in attaching emotional colour to our thoughts and perceptions, and this is indeed the case.

Functional neuroimaging techniques, such as PET, have detected increased activity in the amygdala in sufferers from depression and anxiety (Figure 2.23). In Section 2.4.2 we said that electrical stimulation of the amygdala in humans during brain surgery evokes feelings of heightened dread. In people with depression, the amygdala appears to be unusually active during many tasks. Interestingly, this is true whether the person is currently depressed, or has been depressed in the past and is now in remission. Thus an overactive amygdala may be a marker for the vulnerability to depression rather than just for the symptoms of depression.

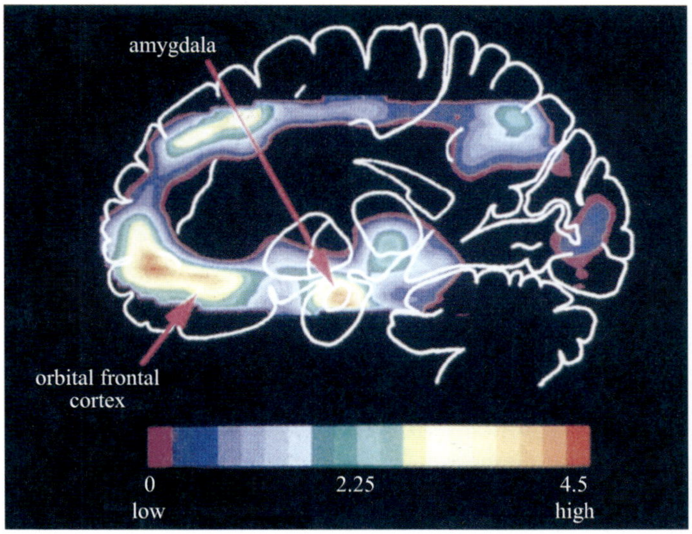

Figure 2.23 Image produced by subtracting PET scans of depressed participants from those of controls. Note the increased activity in the amygdala and the orbital frontal cortex.

- Why might a very active amygdala be related to depression and anxiety?
- Depression involves an excess of the negative emotional associations of any situation. The amygdala is also more active during emotions such as fearfulness and anxiety, and so where its activity is excessive, the person will be quick to respond with these negative emotions.

The amygdala is connected to a network of other areas, all of which may be involved in depression and anxiety. It projects forwards to parts of the frontal cortex. These areas, particularly on the left side, show altered patterns of activity in depressed people when their current state is clinically poor. Thus, if activity in the amygdala is a marker for the vulnerability to depression, the activity in the left frontal lobe may be a marker of the actual state.

Depression is an essentially reversible state, and often arises in people with no prior difficulties of any kind. Symptoms can be successfully reversed, sometimes without any lasting difficulties. Unlike disorders such as schizophrenia (Chapter 3), you would not expect distinct differences in size or shape of brain areas. Nevertheless, there is evidence for cell loss in part of the frontal lobes of depressed patients. The cells that are lost are not neurons, but the supporting glial cells (Book 1, Section 2.4.4). The precise significance of this finding is not yet entirely clear but you have already come across instances of abnormal patterns of functioning that can eventually lead to cell loss or damage of some kind.

In animals who have suffered prolonged anxiety, and in patients with post-traumatic stress disorder, the dendrites in the hippocampus can become shrivelled up, often leading to a significant reduction in its overall size (Figure 2.24). The types of tasks that are impaired by prolonged stress in rats, such as navigating to hidden platforms in a water maze, are just those that depend on the hippocampus. Poor memory often accompanies depression, and since one consequence of excessive life stress can be depression, degeneration of the hippocampus may be a major factor in the associated memory disturbances found after both prolonged stress and depression.

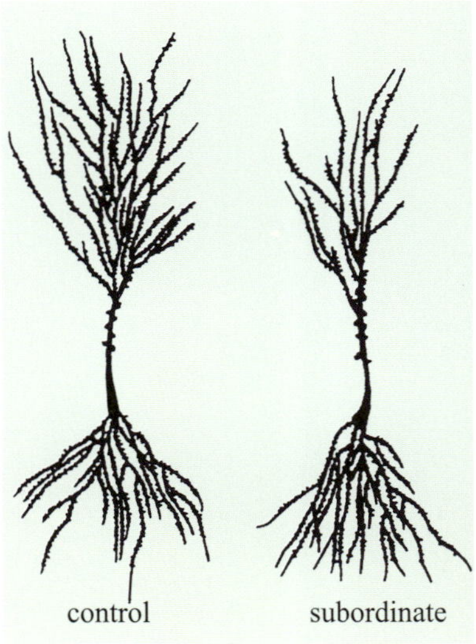

Figure 2.24 Dendrites shrivelled by social stress. Neurons are shown from unstressed (control) and stressed tree shrews (*Tupaia belangeri*), a mammalian species related to early primate evolution.

2.12 Genetic influences on affective disorders

In Book 3, Section 3.9 you saw how genetic factors (and environment) can influence violent behaviour. Similarly, genetics are thought to be important in both individual differences in emotional reactions, and in a range of emotional disorders. In rodents (Gray, 1987), there are clear genetic differences among individuals in reactivity and learning about fearful stimuli.

For example, Figure 2.25 shows the effect of 30 generations of selective breeding in mice for high and low activity in the Open Field (compared with unselected controls). The continuing divergence in fearful behaviour between the selective groups suggests that many genes are likely to be responsible for this behaviour. If just one or two genes were responsible for Open-Field activity, the high and low activity lines would separate after a few generations and then diverge no further.

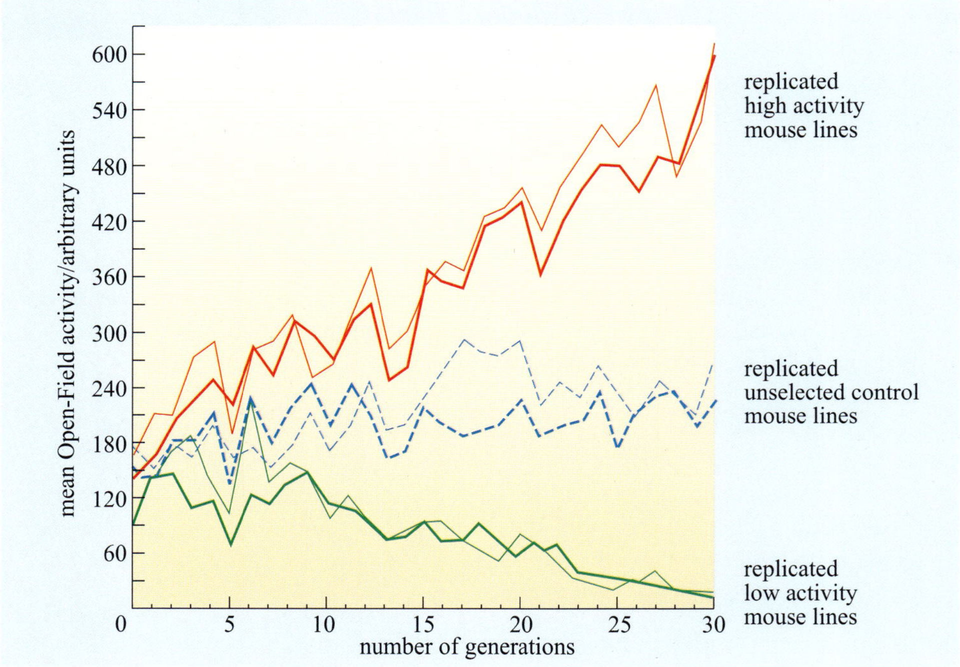

Figure 2.25 Open-Field activity for three strains of mice bred over 30 generations.

Just as with animal models, affective disorders in humans run in families. Concordance rates (the chances that other family members will suffer the same disorder) for both bipolar and unipolar disorders are around 40–50% for monozygotic (genetically identical) twins and 10–15% for dizygotic twins (sharing only, on average, 50% of their genes). The probable influence of genes and environment can be clarified only by adoption studies (think back to the cross-fostering animal studies we have explored earlier). Because these effects remain robust in adoption situations, we can be reasonably sure that genetic factors are involved.

Because temperament and situation interact, temperamental factors (which are partly determined genetically) increase the risk, but the final push into a depressive state comes from situational factors such as stress, bereavement, redundancy, the short day-length seasons, and so on. Changes in society can make these triggers more or less frequent, and thus the rate of depression can change radically without genetic change in the population. The current rising trend is illustrated in Figure 2.26, which comes from a vast American study of the incidence of

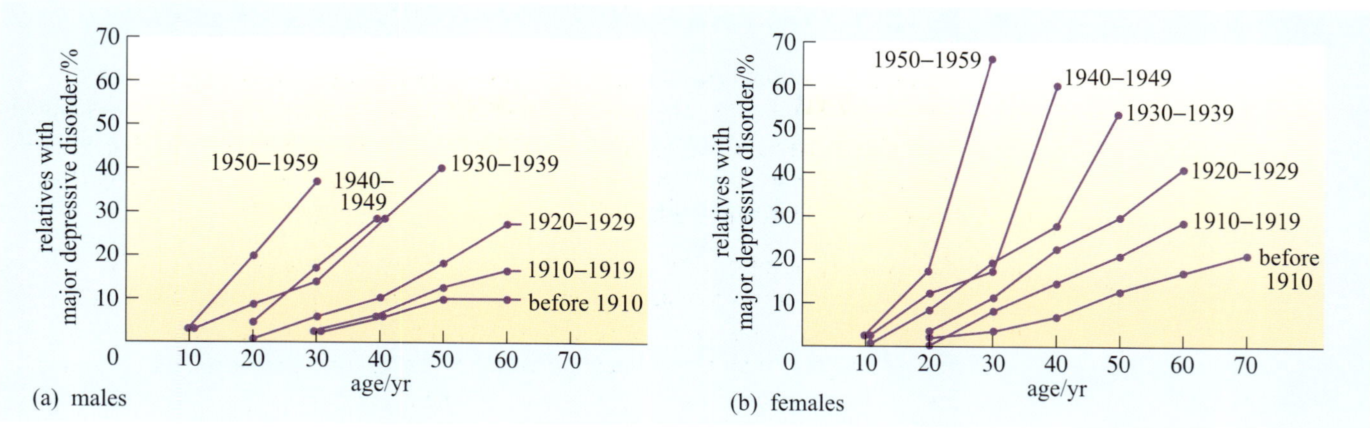

Figure 2.26 Rates of depression in the first-degree relatives of depressed patients, broken down by decade of birth. Note how the rates have increased dramatically through the 20th century, especially among women.

depression in relatives of those with mood disorders. Analysis of the occurrence and co-occurrence of mood disorders such as anxiety and unipolar depression suggest they might have common genetic origins, with the phenotypic differences being dependent on the environment. Thus, for these disorders, situational stresses such as early family dynamics, divorce and bereavement are powerful triggers not just for the occurrence of illness but for the type of disorder that might arise.

2.13 Unipolar and bipolar disorders

Intuitively, it seems likely that unipolar and bipolar depressions are related. After all, the depressive phase of the bipolar form is essentially identical to unipolar disorder. However, anyone who has an episode of mania has a very high probability that both mania and depression will recur throughout their lifespan, whereas a single unipolar episode can disappear never to recur. Bipolar disorder occurs with approximately equal frequency in both sexes, and its incidence is stable. Unipolar disorder, by contrast, affects twice as many women as men, and is, as we have seen, increasing in incidence.

- ◆ From the evidence described above, do you think unipolar and bipolar disorders are the same illness or different ones?
- ◆ They are not identical. Bipolar disorder is probably more strongly controlled by genetic factors, as the stable incidence suggests. It is more intrinsic to the individual, given that its probability of recurrence through life is much higher (or at least was until the advent of lithium as a treatment – see Section 2.14.1). Unipolar disorder is more situationally evoked (although there is a genetic vulnerability), hence the gender imbalance and rising trend.

The above answer might suggest that there is no relationship between the two disorders except for the fact that some of their symptoms happen to be the same. The position is not that clear cut, however. There is familial co-occurrence of the two illnesses, though it is not symmetrical: in the families of bipolar sufferers you almost always find unipolar disorder, whereas in the families of unipolar sufferers you only rarely find bipolar disorder. This may point to different mechanisms for the inheritance of the depressive and the manic/psychotic element of bipolar illness, with the potential for the depressive element, but not the manic element, to be shared with unipolar depression.

2.13.1 Treatments

As we give brief examples of different treatments for emotional disorders, you should see that they neatly highlight the approaches of psychology and biology, and their interactions, which we have taken throughout the course. The more biological approach to treatment targets the chemical environment of the brain, whilst the psychological approach attempts to deal directly with behaviour and patterns of thought. Both approaches are successful, and the optimal strategy is often a combination of the two.

2.14 The chemical approach

Every brain circuit has its characteristic neurotransmitters (Book 1, Section 1.3.2). If one cause of affective disorders is an overactive emotional system, one might expect there to be ways of altering it chemically. This is indeed what antidepressant drugs do. The first antidepressants and antimanic agents were discovered by chance in the 1950s when researchers discovered specific effects on the neurotransmitters **norepinephrine** and **serotonin** (Book 4, Box 1.2). Several studies reveal unusually low levels of chemicals linked to norepinephrine and serotonin in the blood and cerebrospinal fluid of many sufferers from depression. This, coupled with the effects of antidepressants, seems to point to a simple hypothesis – depression is caused by not enough serotonin/norepinephrine being available, or an imbalance of these neurotransmitters.

Of the many types of antidepressants (Table 2.3), some are more specific to serotonin, some to norepinephrine, and some to both. Their action alters the balance or influence of neurotransmitters at the synapse. One class, the **monoamine oxidase inhibitors (MAOIs)** achieves this by disabling an enzyme, monoamine

Table 2.3 Some of the main antidepressant drugs. (Note: you are not expected to remember the names of the antidepressants in this table)

Compound	UK trade name	US trade name
Tricyclics		
Imipramine	Tofranil	Tofranil
Amitrypline	Tryptizol/Lentizol	Elavil/Endep
Nortryptiline	Allegron	Aventyl
Clomipramine	Anafranil	Anafranil
Protryptiline	Concordin	Vivactil
MAOIs		
Phenelzine	Nardil	Nardil
Tranylcypromine	Parnate	Parnate
SSRIs		
Fluoxetine	Prozac	Prozac
Sertraline	Lustral	Zoloft
Paroxetine	Seroxat	Paxil
Fluvoxamine	Faverin	Luvox
Citalopram	Cipramil	Celexa
Venlafaxine*	Efexor	Effexor

*Venlafaxine is a combined serotonin–norepinephrine reuptake inhibitor.

oxidase (Book 3, Section 3.9.2), which is involved in breaking down used neurotransmitter. Another class, the **tricyclics**, works by disabling the chemical pump that reabsorbs serotonin and norepinephrine into the neuron. The **specific serotonin reuptake inhibitors (SSRIs)** do a very similar job but with a much higher specificity for serotonin rather than for norepinephrine. The effects of antidepressants are not simply a matter of replenishing neurotransmitters. Antidepressant drugs increase the amount of serotonin and norepinephrine available at the synapse within a matter of hours of first taking them. The therapeutic effects, though, do not take place until a few days or even weeks later. Post-mortem studies of the brains of suicide victims, many of whom were depressed, suggest an increased abundance of serotonin and norepinephrine receptors in their brains. Thus the therapeutic effect of antidepressants may well be that, by increasing the transmitter present at the synapse, they eventually cause neurons to reduce their excessive production of receptor molecules. Thus the effect is mediated not merely by inputting a chemical for which there may be some shortage, but by inducing change in the neurons themselves.

2.14.1 Bipolar disorder

Unlike the other affective disorders, bipolar disorder is treated with lithium. Treatment begins with antipsychotic drugs during the manic phase. Once mania abates, lithium is generally effective in dampening future cycles of mania and depression. It does, however, have sedating side-effects and is toxic in excessive doses. Cases resistant to lithium can be treated with sodium valproate.

2.15 The psychological approach

In popular imagination, psychological treatments often amount to lying on a couch and relating dreams or childhood experiences that will be interpreted by a therapist in terms of subconscious wishes or desires, often with sexual connotations. Whilst this type of experience could form part of psychoanalytic (such as Freudian) treatment, there are many other approaches. Psychological treatments fall broadly into three different types:

- Those, such as psychoanalytic methods, that seek to unravel the conscious and supposed unconscious origins of distress, and help reduce symptoms by means of analysis and increased awareness of their meaning. Exploration of the style of parenting experienced and relationships with significant family members are a common feature.
- Behaviour therapy, inspired by conditioning theories, that tries to rid the person of the symptoms and behaviour patterns causing distress, without much regard to their origins. Techniques often include using extinction or counterconditioning (new learning that is the 'opposite' of the original, e.g. pairing a pleasant stimulus with something feared or learning to relax in the presence of something feared).
- Cognitive therapy, that attempts to challenge distorted thinking processes and thereby alter some of the automatic assumptions that may arise in emotional disorders.

These latter two methods are often combined into cognitive behaviour therapy.

Box 2.7 Working on biased belief systems in cognitive therapy

In this exchange a therapist is working with a suicidal female client in her mid-twenties. She feels her life is 'worthless' since her husband has taken up with another woman (the therapist is denoted by 'T' and the client by 'C').

C Without Jay I am nothing. I can't live without him, but our marriage can't be saved.

T What has your relationship been like?

C I have been unhappy all along … he is often unfaithful and now we hardly speak at all.

T But you say you can't be happy without him. Are you happy when you are with him?

C No, he puts me down and I feel miserable.

T So you say you are unhappy when you are with Jay? Why do you feel you need your relationship to make you happy?

C I am worthless without him.

T Were you worthless before you met Jay?

C No.

T And were you happy before you met?

C Yes.

T So you have been happy without Jay.

C Yes.

T Did you have male friends before you knew Jay?

C Yes, I was pretty popular.

T And have any men shown an interest in you recently?

C Yes, sometimes they do but I'm married so I ignore them.

T Do you think they would continue to be interested if you were available?

C Yes, I suppose so.

T Do you think there are men who are as good as or better than Jay who might be interested in you?

C Yes.

The interchange continues until the client comes to believe that logically she would be better off leaving her husband and starting out afresh. As a result of the therapy she came to view her marriage as something that was already dead and that there were other options open to her. The notion that 'unless I am loved I am worthless' passed.

Box 2.7 includes a hypothetical extract from a treatment session in cognitive therapy. The therapist seeks to challenge the client's assumptions regarding her relationship with her husband. By exposing some of the irrational conclusions that the client has reached regarding how her happiness is determined by being loved by her husband, the therapist tries to encourage her to consider alternative interpretations of the situation, and thereby new choices of action for the future.

To provide an example of how cognitive behaviour therapy can work, think back to our earlier discussions, e.g. Section 2.7 and Figure 2.19, where we explored how emotional response are elaborated by detecting and appraising any physiological responses to the situation. What happens if this appraisal becomes distorted? Figure 2.27 outlines Clark's (1986) model of what might happen in panic disorder, and is based on the patients' own reports of panic attacks. They may interpret, for instance, a racing heart as indicating imminent catastrophic

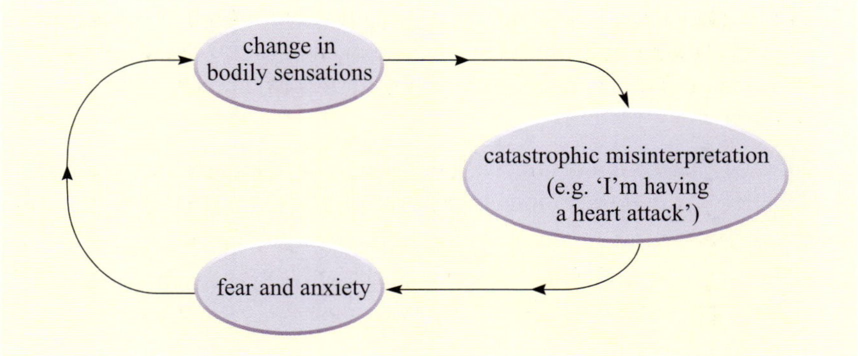

Figure 2.27 Clark's cognitive model of panic. The model suggests that during panic the sufferer experiences physiological responses as a result of an event (this could be exertion from exercise, or a mildly emotional situation) but misinterprets them as indicating illness or even the onset of a life-threatening event such as a heart attack. In turn this elicits fear, thus magnifying the physiological response, further exacerbating their distress in a rapidly escalating vicious cycle – a catastrophic misinterpretation of physiological responses.

consequences such as 'I'm about to have a heart attack'. Not surprisingly, this creates fear, further increasing heart rate and the urgency of the interpretation in a vicious cycle. (Clark (1986) assumes that these types of interpretation may become so fast and automatic that they fail to reach conscious awareness.) Patients often develop coping strategies that include avoiding anything, such as excitement or exercise, which might increase their heart rate. These strategies can severely limit the patients' lifestyle as they maintain a constant anxiety that only by careful behaviour can they avoid a cardiac arrest. This avoidance, of course, prevents them from discovering that the racing heart was in fact innocuous. Treatment involves promoting the alternative appraisal that a racing heart can come from exercise or excitement and need not indicate heart problems, and that even quite strenuous exercise (and increased heart rate) does not have adverse consequences.

Variants such as controlling the method of thinking rather than the contents of thoughts, such as **mindfulness-based cognitive therapy (MBCT)** (Box 2.8), have proved successful in, for example, depression. Conventional cognitive therapy might proceed by challenging a depressogenic thought such as 'I am a complete failure, I'll never be any good at anything' and persuading a patient to recognize this as a distortion and overgeneralization. Mindfulness-based cognitive therapy, by contrast, emphasizes a mental shift, and tries to encourage patients to consider thoughts and feelings as mental events, rather than accepting or trying to deal with

Box 2.8 Mindfulness-based cognitive therapy (MBCT)

Mindfulness means paying attention in a particular way – on purpose, in the present moment and non judgementally.

Cognitive therapy aims to teach patients to change the content of their negative thoughts. It is better than 'clinical management' for preventing relapse but requires 16–20 hours of individual therapy.

In MBCT, there is little emphasis on changing the content of thoughts. Rather, patients are systematically trained to be more aware, moment by moment, of thoughts, feelings and physical sensations – there is a shift to a decentred relationship to thoughts and feelings – these are seen as passing mental events, not 'me', not 'facts'. Integrating mindfulness training and cognitive therapy, opens up a new strategy for treating a wider range of disorders.

In a trial, depressed patients who had suffered from a recurrent series of depressive episodes were randomly allocated either to receive MBCT or to continue their regular treatment as usual. For patients with three or more previous episodes, MBCT can halve relapse for an investment of less than three hours' instructor time per patient (Figure 2.28).

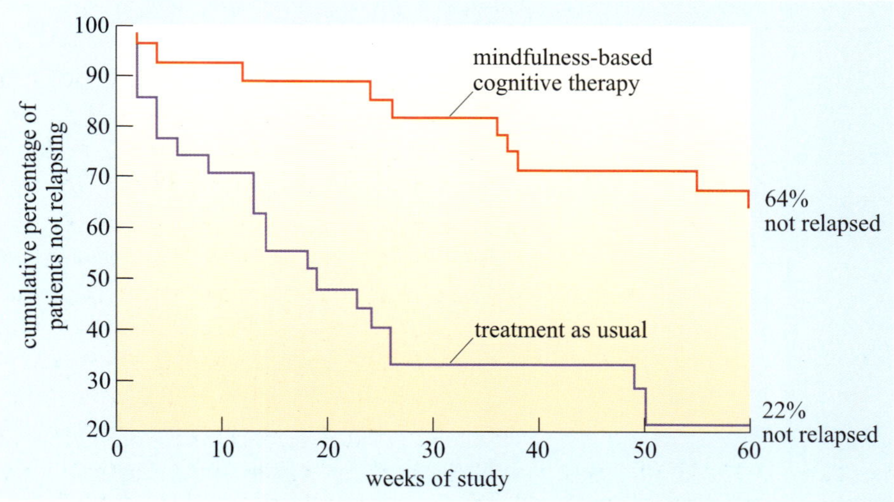

Figure 2.28 Graph showing the results of a treatment trial comparing mindfulness-based cognitive therapy with previous treatment as usual. At the beginning of the trial all participants were in remission. Over the next 60 weeks they were followed up to check whether they were still free of depression. From the graph it is clear that MBCT slows down or even prevents relapse into another depressive episode over the time-course of the trial.

or modify their meaning. In the above example they might think: 'At this moment I'm having a thought that I am a failure... This is a thought and is not a fact. Having a thought that I am a failure does not mean that I am a failure'.

Controlled studies show that some forms of psychotherapy can be about as effective as drugs. The optimal strategy is often a combination, with drugs to break the immediate negative spiral, and psychotherapy to identify and avoid troublesome psychological patterns and associations, and to help prevent relapse without the need for lifetime drug dependence.

A number of controlled studies have shown that drugs can alter the types of attitudes that are prevalent in depression. Some examples of these, so-called, dysfunctional attitudes can be seen in Box 2.9, which provides an extract from the type of dysfunctional attitude scale used in the experiment. Figure 2.29 shows the change in scores brought about by receiving either a single dose of an antidepressant or a control drug. Thus drugs can clearly influence distressing thoughts and thereby relieve symptoms of emotional disorders. Brain-imaging studies show that cognitive appraisal, such as deliberately thinking about material in an emotional or objective style, alters brain activation.

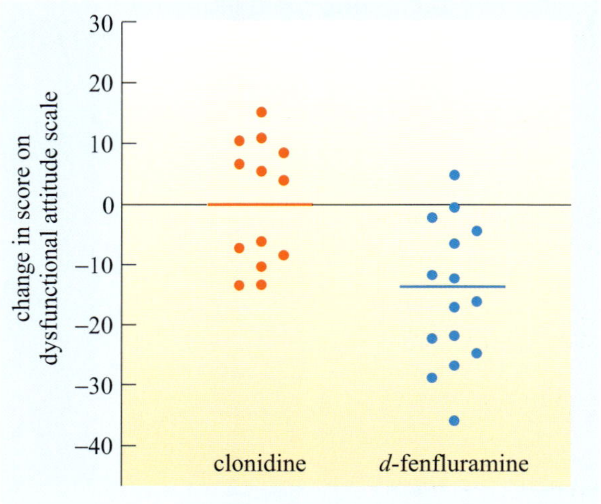

Figure 2.29 Change in dysfunctional attitude scale scores for 28 healthy participants after a single dose of either intravenous *d*-fenfluramine (an antidepressant drug) or clonidine (control drug). Note: red and blue lines indicate mean values.

- ◆ The effectiveness of antidepressant drugs seems to show that depression is a chemical imbalance, whereas the effectiveness of psychotherapy seems to show that it is in the mind rather than in response to chemicals. Which is it?

- ◆ Depression is both in the mind and a chemical imbalance. Brain activity on the one hand, and thoughts and feelings on the other, are not two separate items but different aspects of the same highly complex phenomenon. Psychological disorders represent imbalances at every level from the molecule to thoughts and feelings, and successful intervention will interactively affect all of those levels.

- ◆ Psychotherapy is not usually the first intervention in acute mania. Why do you think that this might be?

- ◆ Psychotherapy requires the patient to see that there might be patterns of thought and behaviour worth changing. In depression and anxiety, thoughts and behaviour are causing unhappiness, so the person is quite likely to seek change. In mania, which by definition involves great confidence and euphoria, the person is unlikely to see any problem, despite the danger of the condition.

Box 2.9 Dysfunctional attitudes

Holding so called 'dysfunctional attitudes' is a hallmark of mental disorders such as depression. A dysfunctional attitude scale includes items similar to those below. Individuals are asked to rate how much they agree or disagree with each statement and their answers are totalled to give a dysfunctional attitude scale score.

	Agree strongly	Agree slightly	Neutral	Disagree slightly	Disagree strongly
1 I need other people's approval in order to be happy					
2 If I fail at work, then I am a failure as a person					
3 If I strongly believe I deserve something, I have reason to expect that I should get it					
4 If a person asks for help it is a sign of weakness					
5 If a person I love does not love me, it means I am an unlovable person					
6 If a person avoids problems, the problems tend to go away					
7 Happiness is more a matter of my attitude towards myself than the way other people feel about me					
8 It is possible to gain another person's respect without being especially talented at anything					
9 Making mistakes is not necessarily bad as I can learn from them					
10 I do not need the approval of other people in order to be happy					
11 If someone disagrees with me it does not necessarily mean they dislike me					
12 I can find happiness without being loved by another person					

Scoring: For the first 6 items, a tick in the 'agree strongly' box would result in a score of 5 for each item, a tick under 'agree slightly' gains a score of 4, and so on. For the last 6 items, agreeing with the statement is less dysfunctional than agreeing. For items such as these, scoring would be reversed and a score of 5 would be given for each 'disagree strongly' answer, and a score of 1 for each 'agree strongly' answer, and so on. The items have been grouped together for clarity in this example, but would normally be randomly organized to avoid a bias of responding at one end of the scale or the other.

Summary of Sections 2.14 and 2.15

Treatment of emotional disorders can involve drugs that influence brain chemistry, particularly those targeting serotonin and the serotonin receptors. Psychological methods can achieve success by 'listening therapy', conditioning new behaviour, or by altering the way a patient thinks about the distressing situation or their past experiences. Combined methods can be particularly effective when initial states are severe or resistant to initial treatment. Drug treatments influence cognitive appraisal of emotional situations and likewise cognitive appraisal alters brain activity.

Learning outcomes for Chapter 2

After studying this chapter you should be able to:

2.1 Recognize definitions and applications of each of the terms printed in **bold** in the text.

2.2 Outline the range and universality of different emotions.

2.3 Reflect on the evolutionary function of emotions.

2.4 Provide an overview of the main brain areas and pathways implicated in emotion.

2.5 Outline some features of emotional disorders and their treatments.

2.6 Demonstrate an understanding of some emotional disorders and types of treatments.

2.7 Contrast cognitive and neurobiological models of fear and anxiety.

Questions for Chapter 2

Question 2.1 *(Learning outcome 2.2)*

Which emotion expressions have emotion researchers generally considered to be pan-cultural when they have tried to test the universality of emotion expressions? What experimental techniques have these researchers used in their investigations?

Question 2.2 *(Learning outcome 2.3)*

When the emotion of fear leads to a physiological response in the body, what general effect does this have on the way we are able to respond, and what evolutionary function might this serve?

Question 2.3 *(Learning outcome 2.4)*

Which of the following pathways provides the 'quick and dirty' route that gives rise to an emotional response for fear, and which gives rise to the slower, more precise route for the same emotion?

A thalamus → amygdala → emotional response

B amygdala → cortex → hippocampus → emotional response

C thalamus → cortex → amygdala → emotional response

D spinal cord → basal ganglia → cerebellum → emotional response

Question 2.4 *(Learning outcome 2.4)*

Which area of the brain is sometimes called the 'hub of the wheel' in emotion research?

Question 2.5 *(Learning outcome 2.5)*

According to the 1996 World Health Organisation report, which of the following give(s) rise to more lost life-years than does war?

A unipolar depression

B self-inflicted injuries

C road traffic accidents

D bipolar disorder

Question 2.6 *(Learning outcome 2.5)*

Which of the following symptoms are included as being important for a diagnosis of depression, according to the American Psychiatric Association?

A insomnia or oversleeping

B persistent feelings of sadness or anxiety

C loss of energy or increased fatigue

D difficulty thinking, concentrating or making decisions

E muscle tension

F restlessness

Question 2.7 *(Learning outcome 2.6)*

Which of the following attitudes might be altered by an antidepressant drug?

A I find the smell of rotting fruit disgusting.

B If a person I love does not love me, it means I am an unlovable person.

C I feel anxious at the thought of going to the dentist.

D I need other people's approval in order to be happy.

Question 2.8 *(Learning outcome 2.7)*

What are the main differences in emphasis between the cognitive and neurobiological approaches to research into the emotion of fear and anxiety?

CHAPTER 3

SCHIZOPHRENIA

3.1 Introduction

As you have gone through this course, you will have gained a sense of the enormous progress that has been made in biological psychology in the last fifty years. We now understand many of the building blocks of the brain, and how these relate to aspects of what we call the mind. But how are these blocks put together? How does an integrated pattern of individual thinking and feeling arise from the chemical and electrical morass of the brain?

One way to approach this question is to ask what happens when thinking and feeling go wrong. They do go wrong; 5–10% of the human population is affected by serious mental illness at some time in their lives, and many more of us have more minor disturbances which prompt us to seek medical attention. Can we understand whence these disturbances come? And if so, what does this tell us about how thinking and feeling are produced in the 'normal' brain?

In this chapter, we will concentrate on one of the most serious, widespread and disabling mental disorders: schizophrenia. This disorder illustrates perhaps better than any other the need to understand the relationship between brain and behaviour at a series of different levels of explanation. Schizophrenia is associated with abnormalities in brain chemicals, neurons, brain anatomy, genes and psychological experience. None of these abnormalities will ever constitute an explanation of schizophrenia until we understand how they relate to each other.

3.2 What is schizophrenia?

J.K.S. was born in Iowa, USA in 1900. She was a competent student who trained to be a teacher, though by her late twenties she did not work. She was highly self-absorbed, sitting for hours on her own, and often giggling privately. In general she was contented, sometimes playful and sometimes apathetic. At the age of 33, she declared her belief that her mother was not really her mother, that she was adopted and possibly had several mothers. This naturally raised concern from her family. Further probing revealed that J.K.S. felt she was being persecuted by a number of people who were using her to make motion pictures. They had concealed cameras in the light fittings and walls, and every time she went somewhere they took footage of her. The directors were constantly pestering her by speaking lines, to which she was forced to respond.

Thus she had been forced to play as Ruby Keeler in the musical *42nd Street*, and in several other movies which were released under the names of Jean Harlow, Joan Crawford and others. The movie organization had even managed to infiltrate the mental hospital to which she was admitted for a month in 1934, placing cameras in 'lightholes'. She received a diagnosis of schizophrenia.

Unusually for a schizophrenia patient at that time, J.K.S. was able to live away from hospital, though she was always dependent on her relatives. She did some driving and shopping. Nonetheless, she intermittently expressed the belief that she was a movie star, and also, later, that she had a large number of children, who were being kept from her by her mother.

The story of J.K.S. illustrates many of the key features of schizophrenia. Contrary to stereotypes (which are largely unfounded in this case), she was not violent or socially irresponsible; nor did she have a 'split personality'. Her abilities to talk, think and carry out everyday tasks were functional and stable. It is just that the content of her thought and speech was so removed from reality that society found it very difficult to relate to her.

Coupled to this was a difficulty in getting on with anything. J.K.S., like many people diagnosed with schizophrenia, would have had trouble holding down a job, or having a relationship, due to a reduced drive to initiate anything and to see it through. Though this was probably tied up with her preoccupation with her strange beliefs, it was not reducible to this. After all, she had been self-absorbed and economically inactive for several years before she reported her strange beliefs to her family and doctors. Schizophrenia is the most troubling of conditions because, reading a case history like this one, we do not know whether to say J.K.S. was ill, or just different from the people around her. We will come back to this issue later in the chapter. What is clear is that J.K.S.'s condition – whether a disease or just a personality trait – meant she lived her life across a deep human chasm from family, society and opportunity for experience.

Around 1% of the human population has been diagnosed with schizophrenia. Though this may seem like a small proportion, it is a huge number for such a profound and lifelong disorder. It equates to 3 million people affected in the United States, and a similar number in the European Union. The human cost of this chronic problem is staggering, since few people recover entirely. J.K.S.'s story is part of a long-term follow-up of people with psychiatric problems in Iowa, USA (Winoukur and Tsuang, 1996). Several decades after diagnosis, of those people with schizophrenia, only around one-third were living independently or with relatives; another third were economically active; a fifth were married. About one-fifth were free of overt psychiatric symptoms. Whichever the professional class people affected by schizophrenia start out in, the usual pattern is for them to drift into unemployment or inability to work. Over the last few decades, the proportion living as hospital inpatients has declined, with more care taking place in the community, but the fundamental outlook, economically, medically and personally, remains very difficult.

3.2.1 Symptoms and diagnosis of schizophrenia

So what exactly is schizophrenia? The concept was proposed by the father of modern psychiatry, Emil Kraepelin, just over one hundred years ago, as a catch-all for psychological breakdowns that arose early in life. The concept has been refined over the years, not least by Eugen Bleuler, who gave it its modern name in 1911. Psychiatrists today use standard lists, such as given in Box 3.1, of the symptoms required for a diagnosis of schizophrenia.

Clinical descriptions divide the symptoms of schizophrenia into positive and negative.

The **positive symptoms** are **hallucinations** (strange perceptual experiences, which can be auditory, visual, tactile or even olfactory), **delusions** (strange and baseless beliefs, often of persecution, special importance or supernatural powers), and **thought disorder**. Thought disorder refers to patterns of reasoning which appear to us to be odd, circuitous, or nonsensical. The positive symptoms are so called because each involves adding something to normal thought patterns.

Box 3.1 Criteria for a diagnosis of schizophrenia

The following list of symptoms required for a diagnosis of schizophrenia is from the American Psychiatric Association's *Diagnostic and Statistical Manual, IV.* (The list is for illustration and you needn't worry about all the terminology at this point.)

A Characteristic symptoms

Two (or more) of the following, each present for a significant portion of time during a 1-month period (or less if successfully treated):

1 delusions

2 hallucinations

3 disorganized speech (e.g. frequent derailment or incoherence)

4 grossly disorganized or catatonic behavior

5 negative symptoms (i.e. affective flattening, alogia, or avolition)

Note: Only one Criterion A symptom is required if delusions are bizarre or hallucinations consist of a voice keeping up a running commentary on the person's behavior or thoughts, or two or more voices conversing with each other.

B Social/occupational dysfunction

For a significant portion of the time since the onset of the disturbance, one or more major areas of functioning such as work, interpersonal relations, or self-care are markedly below the level achieved prior to the onset (or when the onset is in childhood or adolescence, failure to achieve expected level of interpersonal, academic, or occupational achievement).

C Duration

Continuous signs of the disturbance persist for at least 6 months. This 6-month period must include at least 1 month of symptoms (or less if successfully treated) that meet Criterion A (i.e. active-phase symptoms) and may include periods of prodromal or residual symptoms. During these prodromal or residual periods, the signs of the disturbance may be manifested by only negative symptoms or two or more symptoms listed in Criterion A present in an attenuated form (e.g. odd beliefs, unusual perceptual experiences).

D Schizoaffective and Mood Disorder exclusion

Schizoaffective Disorder and Mood Disorder With Psychotic Features have been ruled out because either (1) no Major Depressive Episode, Manic Episode, or Mixed Episode have occurred concurrently with the active-phase symptoms; or (2) if mood episodes have occurred during active-phase symptoms, their total duration has been brief relative to the duration of the active and residual periods.

E Substance/general medical condition exclusion

The disturbance is not due to the direct physiological effects of a substance (e.g. a drug of abuse, a medication) or a general medical condition.

F Relationship to a Pervasive Developmental Disorder

If there is a history of Autistic Disorder or another Pervasive Developmental Disorder, the additional diagnosis of Schizophrenia is made only if prominent delusions or hallucinations are also present for at least a month (or less if successfully treated).

The **negative symptoms**, by contrast, all involve a reduction in some normal activity. They include flattened affect (a reduction of normal emotional reactions), reduced motor activity and fluency of speech, alogia (reduced fluency of thought), and avolition (difficulty initiating things by one's own will power).

The exact combination of positive and negative symptoms observed varies from case to case, but a positive symptom such as hearing voices is given special significance in the diagnosis. Positive symptoms are also called psychotic symptoms. **Psychosis** is any severe mental illness in which there is a break from reality, and positive symptoms constitute such a break.

Despite this clear description, it is fair to say that the unity of the disorder is still questioned in various quarters. The problem is twofold; the diversity of symptoms that can be present, and their lack of specificity. Apart from J.K.S., no other patient, of the hundreds of millions who have had schizophrenia has ever had the precise delusion of being forced to play Ruby Keeler in *42nd Street*. One might say that that is unimportant: what unifies the disorder is that *some* unusual belief or experience is present. Here we encounter the specificity problem, though. Strange beliefs and experiences are quite common in mania and depression, in acute brain damage, in certain types of epilepsy, and in stages of Parkinson's disease. In fact, studies show that occasional hallucination is moderately common amongst people who do not come under medical attention at all.

This type of consideration makes it attractive to argue that those diagnosed with schizophrenia have nothing at all in common except that their beliefs are too different for society to accept them, and nothing else can be found to be wrong with them. This kind of argument was influential, particularly in the 1960s, when authors like Thomas Szasz claimed that schizophrenia was not a disease at all, but rather a label applied by the social system on those it sought to marginalize (Szasz, 1974). This is what is called a *constructionist argument*. Constructionist views see entities like diseases as products of our ways of talking about and classifying the world. A constructionist approach to schizophrenia would see it as a category created by doctors and society, and not primarily something which actually exists in the brain. The apparent validity of a concept like schizophrenia is partly a self-fulfilling prophecy. If you treat someone as unusual or disordered, then before long they may start to behave in a disordered way in response to the application of that label.

Constructionist arguments were relatively popular twenty or thirty years ago, before the biology underlying schizophrenia began to be understood. Interest in them has tended to wane as explanations in terms of the brain have started to be supported by the evidence. However, the constructionist argument has some important lessons which remain relevant as we interpret the biological evidence, as we will do in this chapter. In particular, the constructionist approach raises issues to do with the boundary between different disorders, and between disorder and normality, which remain important, as we shall see in Section 3.6.

3.2.2 From symptoms to prodromes: the neurodevelopmental hypothesis

As already mentioned, the psychotic symptoms of schizophrenia, hallucinations and delusions, generally come on in adolescence or young adulthood. They may then become chronic, or they may remit quite quickly, with or without later recurrence. However, it is very clear from case studies like that of J.K.S. that the problems faced by people with schizophrenia do not begin and end with delusions and hallucinations. J.K.S. already had difficulties of integration into social and economic life several years before reporting her strange beliefs.

Descriptions of schizophrenia report social withdrawal and problems of coordination, attention, concentration and willed action. These problems form the enduring underscoring of a life punctuated by episodes of psychotic symptoms. The subtle, ongoing difficulties are often ignored in popular descriptions of schizophrenia, since the psychotic symptoms seem so much more dramatic. Nonetheless, the evidence is mounting that they may be just as important.

Patients with schizophrenia show performance difficulties on many tasks. In IQ tests, the distribution is shifted several points downwards compared to that of the normal population, and indeed, on a wide variety of pen and paper or practical problem-solving tasks, patients have a deficit. They show particular problems when they have to keep focused attention on one element of a display, or ignore irrelevant or distracting information in order to complete a task. These psychological difficulties can be picked up at a very biological level. Over 80 studies have shown that schizophrenia patients have abnormal patterns of eye movements when following a target or scanning a display (Figure 3.1). The responses of their brains, as estimated by the patterns of minute electrical activity across the scalp (EEG), are also unusual. In one well-studied paradigm, they do not seem to get used to a repeated signal as quickly as control participants do, continuing to show a large cortical response to it even after several repetitions. In another EEG paradigm, participants have to look out for a relevant signal (a high tone) amongst a series of irrelevant ones (low tones). Schizophrenia patients tend not to show such a strong increase in response when the relevant signal comes along. It seems there is a profound problem with paying and keeping selective attention.

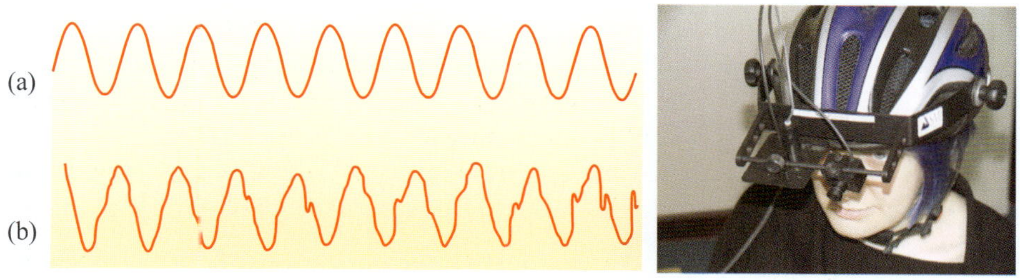

Figure 3.1 The eye movements of (a) a normal volunteer and (b) a person with schizophrenia in following a smoothly moving target on a screen. The photograph shows an example of the apparatus used to track eye movement.

- What do you think the relationship might be between the psychotic symptoms of schizophrenia and the problems with tasks requiring selective attention? How would you test whether your answer was correct?

- There are several possible relationships. First, the problems with selective attention could be the result of having psychotic symptoms. It must be very distracting to have voices going on in your head, or even the fear that such voices might start up. Second, cognitive impairments could cause psychotic symptoms. Third, both psychotic symptoms and cognitive impairments could be the result of a disease process which is not itself directly detectable. You could test between the first and second of these possibilities by looking at the timing of onset; which appears first, the cognitive impairments or the psychotic symptoms? Do the cognitive impairments reduce when the psychotic symptoms are in remission?

As you will have seen from the above question, the question of timing seems critical – do cognitive impairments precede or follow the onset of psychotic symptoms? The answer to this question was difficult to discover for many years, since people with schizophrenia only come to the attention of doctors and researchers once psychotic symptoms occur. However, there are various sources of information which researchers have managed to use to delve back into the past.

Some countries have systems of compulsory military service. Upon entry into the army, young people take a wide variety of psychological tests. If some of them later develop schizophrenia, researchers can refer back to their test results. This strategy has been used by a group from Tel Aviv University on an Israeli sample (Davidson *et al*., 1999). They found that those people who would go on to receive a diagnosis of schizophrenia did worse than their peers on tests designed to measure intelligence, social functioning, organizational ability, autonomy and interest in physical activity. Britain does not have compulsory military service, but it has on several occasions run national surveys of child development. Once again, these can be referred back to if some participants can be identified who later developed schizophrenia. This time the information comes not from age 18 as in the Israeli sample, but from much earlier in life. Research teams led by Peter Jones and Tim Crow found that those people who would go on to be diagnosed with schizophrenia learned to walk and talk slightly later, did a little worse on school tests at 7, 11 and 15 years, were more likely to be socially anxious and to prefer solitary play, and were more likely to be considered as clumsy than were control children. (Some examples are shown in Table 3.1.)

Table 3.1 Comparisons of those who will go on to be diagnosed with schizophrenia and controls, on various developmental measures, from Britain's National Child Development Studies.

	Controls	Patients who would later develop schizophrenia
Early childhood		
age at standing/months	11.4	11.6
age at walking/months	13.5	14.7
age at talking/months	14.3	15.5
7 years		
reading test score	23.3	18.4
mathematics test score	5.2	3.9
11 years		
intelligence test score	43.2	33.2

Source: adapted from Jones *et al.* (1994); Crow *et al.* (1995).

Another, ingenious experimental method used by Elaine Walker and her colleagues reveals how dramatic these early-life difficulties are (Walker and Levine, 1990). They studied the home movies shot in all innocence by the families of those who were later diagnosed with schizophrenia, and those who were not. Skilled observers who did not know the later outcome could easily identify those who would later develop schizophrenia in the great majority of cases, just from their spontaneous motor and social behaviour on the films. This applied to children in their first few years of life who would not experience positive symptoms for another two decades.

The EEG and eye movement tasks have not yet been administered to children. However, they have been administered to the close relatives of schizophrenia patients. These relatives show some degree of impairment, whether or not they have (yet?) developed psychotic symptoms themselves. All this evidence suggests strongly that there is a developmental pathway to psychosis, which begins quite early on with motor, cognitive and social difficulties. If the pathway is followed without interruption, it can eventually lead to psychotic symptoms. Biological relatives show some signs of being on or close to the pathway, though they may not go all the way down it themselves.

This view is called the **neurodevelopmental hypothesis of schizophrenia**. It was developed in the 1980s, and has been very influential, because it radically shifts the way we think of the disorder. Perhaps psychosis is not the iceberg but just the tip – the bizarre extreme state of a problem with the development of the nervous system which has been going on for decades and causing subtler but nonetheless significant difficulties all that time. Under this view, the early-life problems are just as much part of the syndrome as psychosis is. In fact, they have a special place, because they are an early warning sign of the path the patient is on. In medical parlance, they are **prodromal** symptoms; symptoms that give prior warning of others that may follow later. The prodromal symptoms are of special interest, since tackling the problem at that stage might allow us to arrest the disorder's development before it has gone too far. To do that, though, we need to understand what in the brain causes this abnormal trajectory of neural development in the first place.

3.3 The brain basis of schizophrenia

The founders of psychiatry, like Emil Kraepelin, believed firmly that they were dealing with a biological disorder when they delineated the syndrome of schizophrenia. It was soon discovered, though, that unlike cases of aphasia (Book 5, Sections 2.3.2 and 2.3.3) where post-mortem investigation of the brain showed a particular region of the cerebral cortex to be knocked out, there was no brain damage visible to the naked eye at post-mortem in schizophrenia. In the middle part of the 20th century, explanations for psychological disorders focused strongly on social explanations, and it was common to argue that the factors relevant to schizophrenia were to be found in patterns of family relationships rather than in biology. In fact, the evidence for the idea that parenting is at fault in schizophrenia was never impressive. Rather, it was something that was accepted as part of the general assumptions of the times. Even if parenting had been shown to be unusual, of course, it would not prove that odd parenting caused schizophrenia. It could equally be the case that odd parenting was a *response* to a child who showed unusual thought and behaviour.

- ◆ If schizophrenia were caused by patterns of parenting (as was argued in the 1950s) would this make the search for a basis in the brain irrelevant?
- ◆ Explanations in terms of parenting and explanations in terms of the brain are not mutually exclusive. Whatever the factors are that bring schizophrenia on, they must have a seat in the brain. If parenting is at fault, then that parenting will affect the brain (most probably through stress hormones, which are elevated by psychological conflict, and which in turn affect several structures and chemicals within the brain). The search for biological mechanisms is therefore equally relevant if schizophrenia has social causes as if it has genetic ones.

A revolution in our understanding of schizophrenia began, slowly at first, in the 1950s. First, drugs were discovered which were of use in treating schizophrenia. Then more information about how those drugs worked became available. Early forms of brain scan showed up abnormalities deep in the brain that were not visible from the outside. More recently, PET and MRI scanning (Book 3, Section 2.4.1) have provided more detailed evidence concerning brain structure and functioning. Nonetheless, it is still often said that we do not yet know what the brain basis of schizophrenia is. We will see that this is not because of a shortage of candidates. The abnormalities that have been found are measurable at several different levels; the level of brain chemicals (neurochemical level), the level of brain cells, i.e. neurons (cellular level); the level of brain structure (neuroanatomical level); and the level of brain functioning.

3.3.1 The chemical level

The first psychiatric drugs came into use in the 1950s. They were a class called the **phenothiazines**, and they were found to reduce hallucinations and delusions in patients reporting these symptoms. Their discovery was quite accidental; one was derived from a plant which was considered in traditional Hindu medicine to be good for insomnia, whilst the other was intended to be an antihistamine! The phenothiazines quite quickly became the mainstay of treatment for chronic schizophrenia. Further research showed that they inhibit the activity of dopamine, the brain neurotransmitter, which had only just been discovered (Book 4, Box 1.2). (You will learn more about this mechanism in Section 3.5.)

Drugs of abuse like cocaine and amphetamine, on the other hand, increase the activity of brain dopamine (as we saw in Section 1.4.4), and they can cause episodes of hallucinations, delusions, and paranoia when taken by otherwise normal individuals. These observations led to the formulation of a simple neurochemical hypothesis for the mechanism of schizophrenia: that there is an excess of dopamine activity in the schizophrenic brain.

- ◆ Without yet having reviewed the evidence below, and using just what you have learned of schizophrenia so far in the chapter, can you think of any conceptual problems with this dopamine hypothesis?

- ◆ The dopamine hypothesis could be an explanation of schizophrenia if we took delusion/hallucination and schizophrenia to be synonymous. Phenothiazines do suppress hallucinations, and cocaine and amphetamine can cause them. However, phenothiazines have little effect on negative symptoms, or the difficulties with cognitive and attentional tasks. (In fact, due to side-effects, they can even make these symptoms worse.)

At the time the dopamine hypothesis was formulated, researchers assumed hallucination and delusion to be the core of the disorder. Nowadays, however, we believe that they may be more the tip than the iceberg. The difficulties of motor coordination, social behaviour and cognitive development can be evident at least twenty years before the onset of psychotic symptoms, and endure when those psychotic symptoms remit. The dopamine model is really a model of the psychotic symptoms of schizophrenia, not of the whole developmental pathway on which those psychotic symptoms may eventually appear. This does not of course mean that it is necessarily wrong; merely that it is perhaps only part of the story.

To test the dopamine hypothesis, you would need to measure levels of brain dopamine. However, there is no way of doing this in the living brain, as the dopamine is distributed in tiny quantities across millions of synapses. The end-product of used dopamine is called homovanillic acid (HVA). HVA is passed from the brain into the blood and cerebrospinal fluid. A sample of cerebrospinal fluid can be taken by a simple procedure called a lumbar puncture, and the HVA levels measured. A high level of HVA indicates a high level of recent dopamine activity. Such investigations, of course, are only of interest in patients who are not taking antipsychotic drugs, because of the known effects of those drugs on dopamine levels.

A few studies using this technique have shown an excess of HVA in schizophrenic patients as compared to controls, but a much greater number have not. One problem in this area is that studies do not clearly separate patients who are currently experiencing psychotic symptoms from those who are not. Given that the dopamine hypothesis only really concerns active psychotic experiences, this is a failing. Nonetheless, overall, there is very little evidence of a general excess of dopamine in the schizophrenic brain.

However, it would be possible for dopamine *activity* to be unusually high without an actual increase in the amount of dopamine in the brain. Every neurotransmitter works in conjunction with a receptor molecule on the other side of the synapse. If the receptor molecules were unusually abundant, for example, a person might become excessively sensitive to dopaminergic activity, even if the actual levels of dopamine present were normal.

There are several methods for studying the abundance of dopamine receptors, of which there are several types, in the brain. The first technique is only possible post-mortem. Brain tissue is bathed in a solution of a radioactively labelled chemical called a ligand which binds to certain dopamine receptors. The excess is then washed off, and slices of the tissue painted with an emulsion that is sensitive to radioactivity. The amount of radioactive ligand left stuck on the brain slice is proportional to the amount of dopamine receptor present. This type of study has generally shown a considerable excess of one type of dopamine receptor (the D2 type) in the brains of deceased schizophrenia patients relative to controls. However, when the comparison is restricted to those who were not taking antipsychotic drugs at time of death, the excess is rather less. Even this may not be a strict enough condition, since those who were drug-free at time of death may nonetheless have had a lot of antipsychotic drugs over their lives, which could have had long-term neurochemical effects.

It is very hard to find a schizophrenia patient who goes right through life without taking any antipsychotic drugs, and this is where the second technique comes in. A participant – alive this time! – is injected with a radioactive ligand for dopamine receptors. He or she then goes into a positron emission (PET) scanner. The amount of ligand retained by different areas of the brain will be related to the abundance of dopamine receptors in that region.

The participants of greatest interest for this technique are those patients who are 'drug-naive', i.e. those who have been diagnosed but not yet received any medication. The first study published showed a clear excess of D2 receptors (Wong *et al.*, 1986; Figure 3.2). However, the second and third studies, using different ligands, showed no significant excess. Subsequent results have been mixed, but it is fair to say that the balance of evidence favours a small but inconsistent increase in D2 receptor density. It may be that the crucial factor in schizophrenia is not the overall density of these receptors, but their distribution across different brain areas.

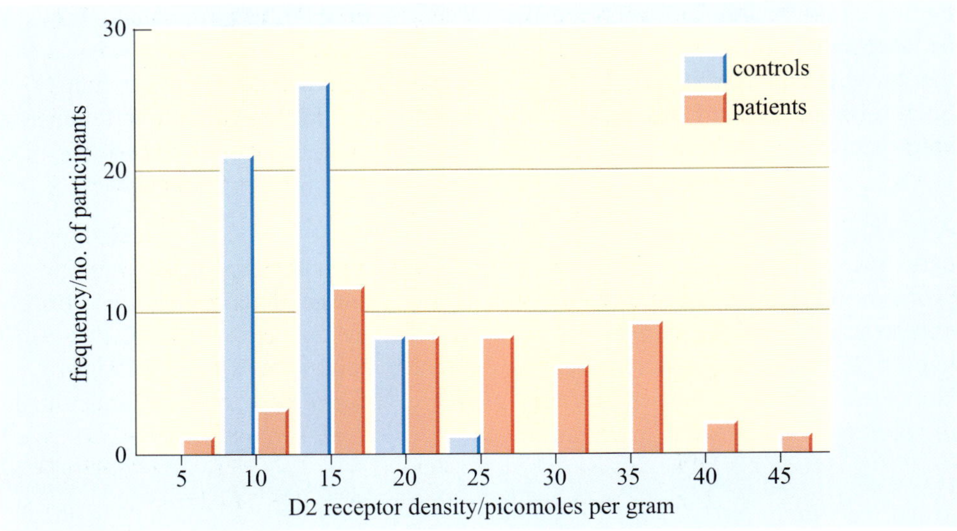

Figure 3.2 Density of D2 dopamine receptors in the putamen of the brains of 56 controls (blue) and 50 schizophrenia patients (red). There are generally much higher densities amongst the patients than the controls, but note the overlapping distributions and the variability within the patients. (You need not worry about the units used in this figure.)

The density of another, very similar dopamine receptor type, D4, has also been studied *in vivo*. Here again, the first published result was positive and caused much excitement, but subsequent studies have shown the evidence for an excess to be weaker and more mixed. Interpretation of the studies is difficult as participants actually experiencing psychotic symptoms are mixed up with those not currently doing so. Overall, though dopamine is clearly often imbalanced in the schizophrenic brain, the abnormality is neither universal nor particularly strong.

There are many neurotransmitters in the brain, each with several types of receptors and a host of supporting chemicals. They are highly interlinked, with cells of one type terminating on those of another, and are similar in their chemical structure. The research focus of neurotransmission in schizophrenia goes on, often with the rationale that somewhere behind the weak and inconsistent dopamine abnormalities is a clearer and more compelling chemical mechanism for the disorder.

Two other neurotransmitters have received special attention. Serotonin (Book 4, Box 1.2) has rather similar claims for attention as dopamine – a hallucinogenic drug of abuse (LSD) is a serotonin agonist (this means it binds to serotonin receptors; see Book 4, Section 1.4.4). Moreover, one class of antipsychotic drugs can be shown to suppress serotonin activity as well as that of dopamine. Serotonin has an important modulatory influence on dopamine activity, so dopaminergic abnormalities might be found even if serotonin was actually the disrupted mechanism (though this may hold the other way around too!). However, there is no evidence whatever that levels of serotonin itself are unusually high in people with schizophrenia. As for the receptors for serotonin, studies have found everything from an excess to a deficiency, and there is no clear pattern overall.

The other neurotransmitter which has been well studied in schizophrenia is glutamate. This is an amino acid which functions as one of the brain's most abundant and widespread excitatory neurotransmitters (Book 4, Box 1.1). Dopamine modulates glutamate release, so there is a link with the dopamine hypothesis (and hence, indirectly, with serotonin too). There is also a drug of abuse – phencyclidine, or PCP – which acts on glutamate receptors and can cause psychotic symptoms. Some post-mortem studies have found a reduction in the amount of either glutamate or its receptors in various critical regions of the brain, such as the hippocampus. However, these studies are at present very inconsistent and find only small effects. The picture is partly complicated by the existence of many different types of glutamate receptor.

It may be that the key chemicals are even deeper in the cellular mechanism. The neuronal membrane itself is formed from fatty acids, and there is some evidence that the metabolism of essential fatty acids is unusual in schizophrenia patients. It has also been found that symptoms improve if the diet is enriched with particular types of essential fatty acids, available through oils extracted from plants or fish. It is even possible that at least some antipsychotic drugs exert their effects, directly or indirectly, on the metabolism of molecules in the cell membrane itself.

Whatever the future fate of these ideas, the picture at the moment is that there are many neurochemical systems that are sometimes or mildly abnormal in the schizophrenic brain, but no single one that can be put forward as a master key. Perhaps the problem is viewing the disorder at the wrong level. Chemical changes in the brain may be fleeting, transitory, and reversible, whereas we saw from the neurodevelopmental evidence that schizophrenia is a lifelong problem not just with hallucination but with coordination, attention and intelligence. Instead of looking for chemical changes associated with the disorder, perhaps we should be looking for structural differences between the brains of schizophrenia patients and the brains of controls at the level of the wiring – that is, of neurons and their circuits.

3.3.2 The cellular level

Some studies have reported finding less grey matter in the brains of schizophrenia patients than controls. Grey matter is the layer, mainly made up cell bodies, that forms the outermost 1 or 2 millimetres of the brain. The difference between grey matter and white matter (the mass of fibres below the grey matter) shows up in an MRI scan. The volume of grey matter can thus be calculated. It is this volume that has been shown to be reduced in schizophrenia patients. Grey matter loss occurs around the time of adolescence anyway, but there is some evidence that this loss is excessive in schizophrenia. Paul Thompson and his colleagues repeatedly scanned young people developing schizophrenia over the course of a five-year period. They found that grey matter loss increased over time, and that the severity of symptoms increased with it (Figure 3.3; Thompson *et al*., 2001).

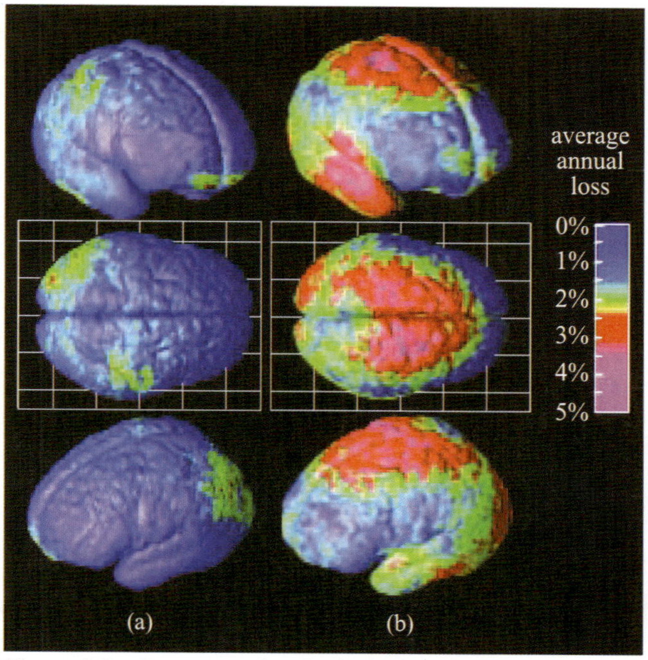

Figure 3.3 Grey matter loss in the brains of young people scanned repeatedly over five years: (a) normal adolescents and (b) those developing schizophrenia. The grey matter loss correlated with a worsening of the symptoms.

This is not the only kind of cellular abnormality found in cases of schizophrenia. Some studies show that the distribution of cells in the cortex into layers is not normal in patients with schizophrenia. The cerebral cortex generally consists of around six layers of cell bodies (Book 1, Figure 3.18). In people with schizophrenia, a greater concentration of cells in the lower layers at the expense of the others has sometimes been observed, though this may vary with different brain regions. The orientation of axons can also be abnormal. One interpretation of these findings is that during early development, as growing cells migrate outwards from their formation in the midbrain to the cortex, their growth gets turned off too soon, resulting in the high concentration in the lower layers of the cortex. As with so much in schizophrenia, the importance of the findings, and the correctness of the interpretation, are not yet clear.

3.3.3 The brain level: structure and function

There is no gross brain abnormality in schizophrenia, but doctors carrying out post-mortems had occasionally observed that the cerebral ventricles, the hollow spaces deep in the brain which in life are filled with fluid, seemed larger than normal. Confirmation of this had to await the development of the first brain scans. In 1976, Eve Johnstone and her colleagues published a paper detailing the use of the early structural brain scanning technique, computerized X-ray tomography (CT) (Book 3, Section 2.4.1). In it, they showed that the cerebral ventricles were indeed enlarged in a sample of schizophrenia patients. (A similar effect is shown in the MRI scan in Figure 3.4.) This result has been replicated many times, and is not a by-product of drug treatment. A couple of points of caution are in order, though. First, patients with other disorders such as manic-depression have enlarged ventricles; and second, there is variability within both the schizophrenic and unaffected populations, with a good deal of overlap between the two.

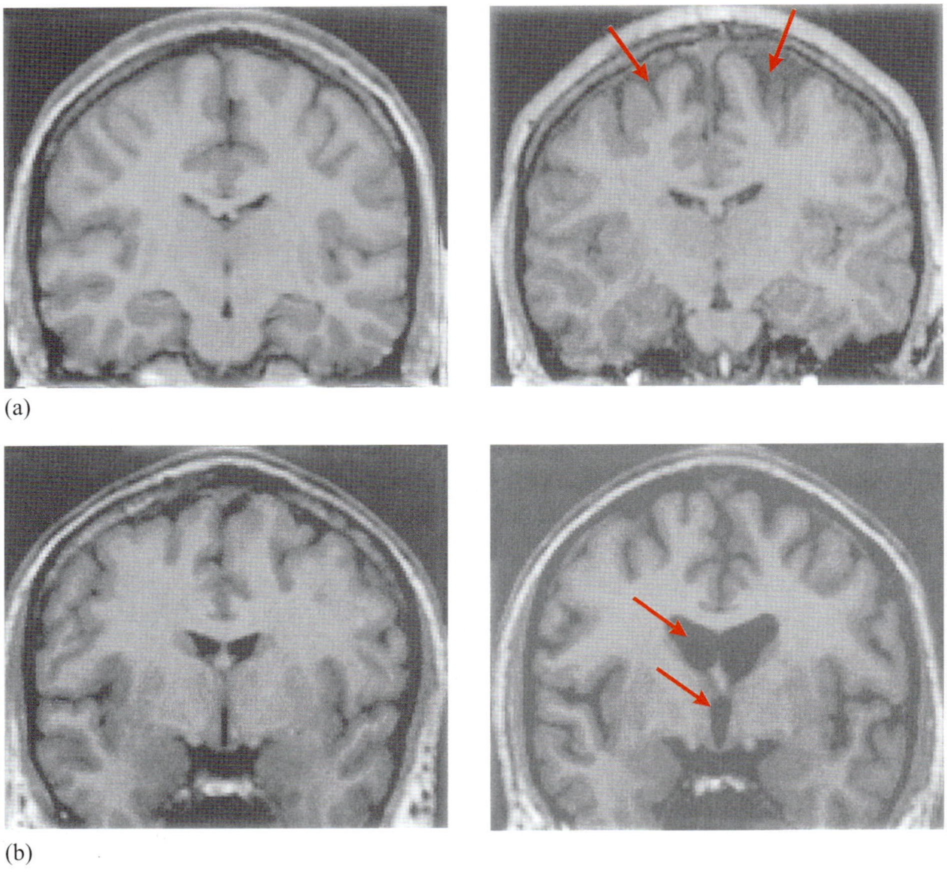

Figure 3.4 MRI scans of control (left) and schizophrenic (right) brains. Note in (a) the thinner layer of grey matter and in (b) the enlarged cerebral ventricles (shown by the arrows).

Enlarged ventricles probably result from loss of tissue in the surrounding midbrain. The CT scanning paper of Johnstone *et al.* (1976) galvanized a whole field of research into the size, shape and composition of the brain in schizophrenia. The findings of differences at this level too have been numerous. First, there are reports that several parts of the brain including the temporal lobes (specifically the hippocampus) and the frontal lobes are smaller than average. All of these findings have been independently replicated, but none of them is a large difference and in all cases the difference is only in the averages of the schizophrenia and control groups. The two groups overlap, so there are many control participants who have smaller brain areas than the schizophrenia groups.

Second, there is evidence for an unusual pattern of asymmetry between the two hemispheres. In most people, the dominant (usually left) cerebral hemisphere is larger and longer than the non-dominant one. In schizophrenia, this pattern is often reduced or non-existent, with the two hemispheres about the same size. Once again, though, the schizophrenia patients sit within the range of variation of the normal population. It is just they tend to be towards the symmetrical end of the distribution.

The third group of abnormalities can be seen not by looking at the structure of the brain, but by watching it in action. This can be done in the PET scanner (see Book 3, Section 2.4.1).

- ◆ How does PET scanning work?
- ◆ Radioactively labelled glucose is injected into the blood. Areas of the brain which are metabolically active pick up more of the glucose than do those parts which are less active. A scanning system placed around the head detects the abundance of the radiation. This is then used to make an image of the brain's activity.

There are abundant differences seen between schizophrenia patients and controls when tasks are performed in the PET scanner. The anatomical location of these differences varies from task to task. The cerebellum is always involved, and the thalamus often is, but otherwise the differences are distributed amongst various regions throughout the brain. There are also differences in the way brain activity shifts. In a task where a normal participant has to make a voluntary (willed), executive decision, perhaps over-riding immediate perceptual responses, there is usually a diversion of blood flow to the frontal lobes, and away from other areas of the cortex. This makes sense, as the non-frontal cortex contains the core areas for immediate sensory interpretation, whilst the frontal lobes are thought to be the seat of complex, planned, voluntary actions (Book 1, Section 4.4.2). Amongst schizophrenia patients, the diversion of blood to the frontal lobe is reduced. The frontal increase is not as large, and the concomitant decrease in other areas is also reduced. Whilst the patient is actually hearing voices, activity is increased in the primary auditory cortex, and when he or she is seeing things, the primary visual cortex is activated (Figure 3.5).

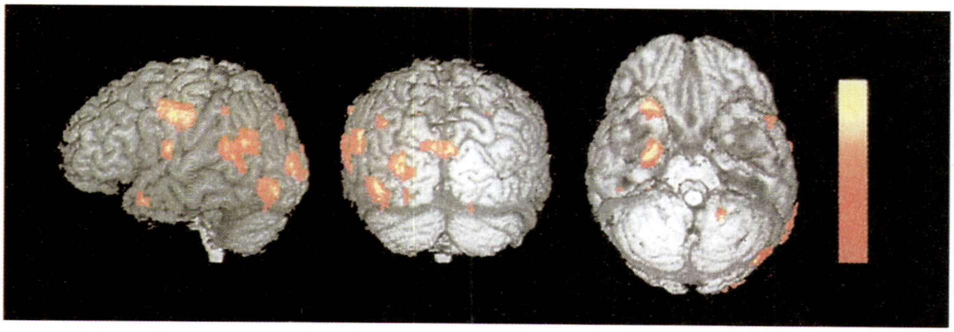

Figure 3.5 PET scans of activity associated with auditory and visual hallucinations in a schizophrenia patient. Many areas of the brain are involved, including parts of the primary sensory areas for vision and hearing. (Red and yellow indicate areas of increased activity compared to controls.)

- ◆ From the information given above, how might you interpret the PET brain activity findings in schizophrenia?
- ◆ The fact that no one area is abnormal suggests that the disorder is to do with how different brain areas connect up, rather than a problem with one specific localized function. The fact that there is activity in the primary auditory cortex during the hearing of voices suggests that the patient really is 'hearing' them in a literal sense.

It makes intuitive sense that no single brain region would be damaged in schizophrenia. After all, memory, language, perception and so on are all basically functional, but their integration into normal mental life is unusual. For this reason, Nancy Andreasen, pioneer of PET studies of schizophrenia, calls the basis of schizophrenia **cognitive dysmetria**, that is, a disorder of the way that cognitive functions integrate (Andreasen *et al.*, 1998). The reduced shifts in brain activity are interesting because they provide a brain correlate of the problems of will and selective attention in schizophrenia. Patients have particular difficulty paying attention to one thing over another, just as they seem to have trouble shifting brain activity from one region to another. If they have trouble shifting activity to their own self-initiated actions, this could explain the negative symptoms of lethargy and difficulty in initiating things.

Summary of Section 3.3 and conclusions

Many types of brain abnormality have been detected in schizophrenia, but they have not always been reliably replicated. At the chemical level, there are increased levels of dopamine receptors. This links to what we know about the functioning of both antipsychotic and hallucinogenic drugs. There is also some evidence for abnormal distributions of serotonin and glutamate receptors, and also that the fatty acids that make up the cell membrane itself are abnormal.

At the neuronal or cellular level, there is evidence that grey matter in many regions of the cortex is thinner in schizophrenia patients than in controls. There is also some evidence that the distribution of cell bodies within cortical layers is unusual, with more cells in the deeper layers and fewer in the surface layers. At the level of the whole brain, there is evidence that the cerebral ventricles are enlarged. Parts of the frontal and temporal lobes are smaller than average, and brain asymmetry may be reduced. Patterns of brain metabolism are unusual in that the regulation of different areas' activity seems to be impaired.

Schizophrenia is a wonderful illustration of the need to understand brain and mind at a series of nested levels. At the highest, psychological level, we have the core problems of cognitive impairment, positive and negative symptoms. The cognitive impairments are probably the key to understanding the other two. Negative symptoms may well be a consequence of the difficulties of attention and shifting activity. Hallucinations and delusions may represent the brain's attempt to interpret abnormal patterns of activity which are going on in unexpected places, like the firing in the auditory cortex when sitting in a silent room. Consciousness gives these a shape and a place in the form of voices.

The psychological manifestations of schizophrenia are underlain by the brain's functioning; the abnormal formation, interconnection and functioning of many different brain regions. These brain-level abnormalities are a product of many billions of cellular abnormalities, which we can partly observe when we look at abnormal axon patterns and grey matter deficiencies. These cellular aberrations are in turn related to chemical imbalances. The causality here could go either way. Abnormal activity of neurotransmitters could lead to cell loss, because neurons that are unable to operate, simply atrophy. On the other hand, the loss of cells and connections could have as a consequence the imbalance of the neurotransmitters that used those cells.

This is all very well, but what is the master trigger in the schizophrenic brain? Of all the many abnormalities we have surveyed, most are at a statistical level only, which means that some patients are more 'normal' on those measures than some people who are diagnosed as healthy. We have an abundance of relative abnormalities, but nothing, as yet, that all and only schizophrenia patients have, which is the master trigger to all the other problems at all the other levels. We will return to this issue in Section 3.6.

3.4 Causes of schizophrenia

If schizophrenia is a disorder of nervous system development, we still need an explanation of why that abnormal development begins. That is to say, dopamine, ventricular enlargement, grey matter thinning and so on are potential mechanisms of the phenomena of schizophrenia, but they are not causes. They must be brought on by some factor or factors. Opinions in this area have followed the general intellectual tide The early 20th century pioneers such as Kraepelin always suspected a genetic factor, even if they did not have the tools to identify it. In the middle of the 20th century, by contrast, people were much more interested in the role of nurture, and in particular relationships between parents and their children.

Contemporary research emphasizes both genetic and environmental factors, as we shall see. Thus both earlier viewpoints have been vindicated to some extent, though the special emphasis on relationship dynamics as causal factors has not been supported by solid evidence.

3.4.1 Genetic factors

The evidence for the involvement of genetic factors comes from family studies, including studies of twins and adopted children. Individuals related to a patient have a much higher risk of developing schizophrenia themselves than do the general population (Gottesman, 1991). The closer the relationship, the higher the risk, as Figure 3.6 shows.

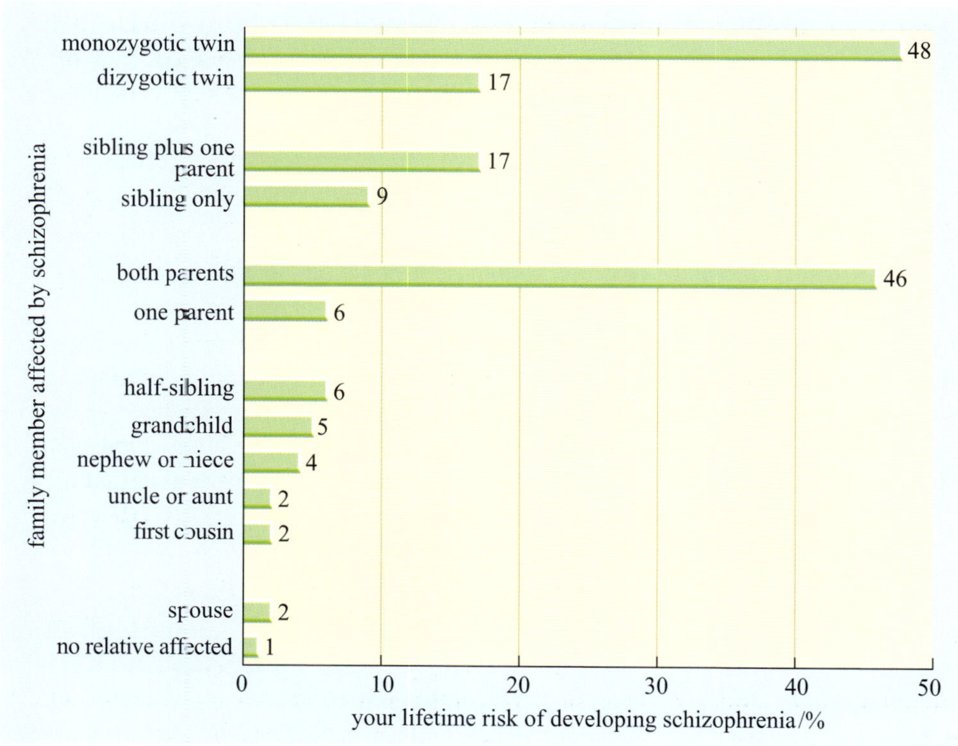

Figure 3.6 Average lifetime risk of developing schizophrenia, estimated from a synthesis of studies of kinship effects.

- ◆ Figure 3.6 shows that schizophrenia runs in families. Does this mean that genetic factors are involved?
- ◆ Not necessarily. Families are also the units of nurture, and share the same environment to a considerable extent. Thus their shared risk for schizophrenia could come from a non-genetic cause.

To test for the relative importance of shared environment and genetic factors, it is necessary to look at twin and adoption paradigms (Book 3, Box 3.2). As it turns out, the degrees of risk for biologically related individuals who are raised apart due to adoption are almost identical to those shown in Figure 3.6, and who have not been adopted. From the dozen or so cases in the literature, we know that where identical twins are raised apart from each other, they are still highly concordant for schizophrenia. There is no evidence that children adopted into a family which contains a schizophrenic member are likely to acquire it. Within biological families, there is a large difference in schizophrenia concordance between monozygotic (identical) and dizygotic (non-identical) twins. It is likely that the environment will be similar for twins whether they are monozygotic or dizygotic; the main difference between them is that the monozygotic twins are much closer genetically than the dizygotic ones (sharing 100% as opposed to 50% of their alleles). Considerations such as these have lead geneticists to estimate that schizophrenia has a **heritability** of about 0.6 in Western societies. (See Box 3.2.)

Box 3.2 Heritability

Heritability is a measure of the extent that variation in a trait is associated with variation in genes. It is expressed as a number between 0 (no association with genetic variation) and 1 (co-varies exactly with genes). Note however that a heritability of 0.6 does not mean that 60% of cases of schizophrenia are caused by genes, or even that a specific individual's illness is 60% due to genes. Every case is caused by genes and the environment in combination. The heritability figure of 0.6 means that, within the study population, 60% of the variation in whether people get schizophrenia is associated with variation in their genes.

This heritability is in some senses an underestimate. The 48% concordance for identical twins counts only those who are diagnosed with schizophrenia, which implies that 52% are free from such problems. In fact, where one such twin is diagnosed with schizophrenia, the other one has some kind of psychological disorder much more often than 48% of the time. The disorder may be a less serious schizophrenia-related disorder like schizotypal personality disorder, or it may have both schizophrenic and other elements – known as a schizoaffective disorder. It may also be a manic-depressive disorder. Thus, the heritability of *some* kind of psychological disorder with psychotic elements is probably rather higher than 0.6.

For a few genetic diseases, like cystic fibrosis, the gene involved has been identified and located. The genetic evidence just presented in the case of schizophrenia suggests strongly that there must be some genetic factor, but it does not tell us which genes are involved. The job of 'gene hunting' is done by scientists using two methods called **linkage studies** and **association studies**. Linkage studies examine the genotypes of all the members of large families which contain individuals both affected and unaffected by schizophrenia. Whatever the genetic factor is, it should more often be carried by the affected than the unaffected members. Any allele significantly more common in the affected group becomes a candidate for checking in other families.

Association studies use large samples of unrelated individuals, again both affected and unaffected by schizophrenia. The logic is similar; alleles that occur significantly more frequently in the affected group become suspects for being involved in the disorder. Association studies have the advantage that large samples can be quickly assembled (since the participants do not have to be related, and can be drawn from the clinical population and general public). However, they have a disadvantage, which is that they can pick up irrelevant differences in the genetic composition of the population. For example, the diagnosis of schizophrenia is more common in urban than rural areas, for reasons that probably have nothing to do with genetics. The urban population has a genetically slightly different composition from the rural one in most countries. For example, the big cities contain more immigrants from other continents, and thus slightly more genetic diversity. An association study might pick up exotic alleles as candidates for involvement in the disorder, where they are in fact irrelevant. Linkage studies do not have this problem, since they hold family background constant by looking at people who are related. Thus the findings of association studies are most convincing when confirmed by linkage within a family.

Many linkage and association studies into schizophrenia have been carried out, and a fair few candidate genes proposed, but many of the proposals have not been supported by subsequent studies. It is fair to say that as yet no gene has been identified whose alleles are unambiguously associated with all or most cases of schizophrenia. This is partly because genetic studies are in their infancy. Another reason is that the liability to schizophrenia is almost certainly a **polygenic trait** rather than a **single-gene trait**.

A polygenic trait differs from a single-gene one in that alleles of more than one gene are involved. Cystic fibrosis (CF) is an example of a single-gene disorder. All individuals affected by CF carry two mutated versions of one particular gene. It doesn't seem to matter what other genes they have; the CF allele is both necessary and (when two copies are present) sufficient for the symptoms to ensue. Polygenic traits are different. Imagine a game of cards, in which the winner was the person who had the Ace of Clubs in her hand. That would be a single-card method of determining who won. An alternative scenario (a polycard game!) would be to count the number of red cards in each player's hand. The one with the most red cards would win. Thus no single red card is either necessary or sufficient for victory; it is to do with how they add up.

Polygenic traits cause problems for linkage and association studies. In our polycard example, if you did a large enough association study, you would not find any one card which was present in all and only winning hands. You would find that all the red cards were more common on average in winning than losing hands, but the difference would be modest. There would be plenty of instances of red cards in losing hands and black cards in winning ones. This is essentially a problem of **statistical power** (Book 2, Section 1.5.3). If a particular card is present in all winning hands and no losing ones, this is such a striking trend that you could detect it using only a sample of a few dozen hands. If a particular card is present in 70% of winning hands and 60% of losing hands, the difference is so subtle that you would need a sample of many thousands of hands to be sure that it really reflected something other than chance. Similarly, polygenic traits require much larger sample sizes for the genes involved to be identified than do single-gene traits. Most heritable characteristics are probably polygenic.

This is one kind of problem hampering the search for genes whose alleles are involved in the liability to schizophrenia. It means that a definitive study will need a massive sample size. There is another problem which has similar effects.

◆ Look again at Figure 3.6. What is the schizophrenia risk for an individual who has an identical twin already diagnosed with the condition? What does this figure tell you about the genetic factor in schizophrenia?

◆ The figure is high (48%), but it is not 100%. Identical twins are in effect genetic clones; their DNA is identical. Therefore, if one twin is sometimes diagnosed with schizophrenia and the other not, there must be non-genetic factors at work too.

Thus, oddly, the genetic research provides the best evidence that we have that the environment is important in the genesis of schizophrenia. The fact that the mapping between genes and the condition is mediated by environmental factors makes gene-hunting even more difficult and requires still larger sample sizes. But what are the environmental factors involved, and how do they operate?

3.4.2 Environmental factors

There is some evidence that those people who undergo a first episode of psychotic symptoms have had a higher than average level of life stressors in the few months prior to the onset. This would also explain why the positive symptoms come on in young adulthood, since levels of stress hormones rise rapidly after puberty. However, the excess of life stress amongst patients is not very great, and it does not distinguish those who will develop schizophrenia from those who will experience depression or anxiety. Moreover, according to the neurodevelopmental hypothesis of schizophrenia, the psychotic episode is just the tip of an iceberg that started to form many years earlier, in the first years of life. Therefore the life stressors just before the breakdown can only really explain why the latent problems got converted into the acute ones at that particular time, not why they exist in the first place. For that, we have to look much further back, in very early development.

There is a modest excess of schizophrenia amongst those born in the winter rather than the summer, and a significant excess in urban and suburban as opposed to rural areas. There is also some evidence that childhood exposure to cats increases the risk a little. Finally, if the mother is infected with a virus such as herpes, rubella or influenza during pregnancy, the risk of later schizophrenia seems to be increased. Table 3.2 shows the **odds ratios** for developing schizophrenia for these four factors. An odds ratio expresses the change in risk of a condition which is brought about by the presence of some factor. For example, if a certain factor increased the risk of schizophrenia from 1 in 100 to 2 in 100, the odds ratio for that factor would be 2.00, (2:100 divided by 1:100). A factor that has no effect at all produces an odds ratio of 1.00 (it doesn't affect the odds). An odds ratio of 1.05 means that the factor increases the risk by 5%. The further away from 1 the odds ratio is, the stronger the effect of the factor.

Table 3.2 Odds ratios for developing schizophrenia for several environmental factors. (Adapted from Heinrichs (2001) and Fuller Torrey *et al.* (2000).)

Factor	Odds ratio
Winter birth	1.05
Urban or suburban residence at birth	1.85
Family owned a cat during childhood (from birth to age 13)	1.53
Mother had any fever during pregnancy	2.82
Complications of birth or pregnancy	1.71

- Look at the first three factors in Table 3.2. How do you think winter birth, urban residence, and exposure to cats might have an effect on the developing nervous system?
- The most likely answer is through infectious disease. There will be more viruses around in winter than in summer, in crowded urban rather than rural areas, and many viruses come to humans through domestic animals. Thus the three apparently different factors are probably all related.

Complications of pregnancy and birth also increase the risk of schizophrenia, particularly those which are likely to lead to nutritional stress or a lack of oxygen supply to the fetus or baby. This is shown in the fifth factor in Table 3.2. None of these effects is dramatically strong; there are many people born on a June day to a healthy mother with no apparent difficulties who still develop schizophrenia. What is more, the factors are probably not sufficient to cause the condition on their own; rather, they interact with a genetic vulnerability. Nonetheless, they do show how environmental disruptions to the delicate young nervous system are a significant step down the path to schizophrenia.

Summary of Section 3.4 and conclusions

Family and adoption studies demonstrate that there is a genetic factor in the vulnerability to schizophrenia. However, due to the polygenic and multifactorial nature of the condition, genetic studies have been unable as yet to unambiguously identify the genes involved.

Genetic factors interact with environmental ones. Early-life factors increasing the risk include winter birth, maternal infection with a virus, and obstetric complications. Later in life, actual episodes may be set off by life stresses, the process of maturation, or drugs.

We have, then, a picture of multiple levels of causation. It is probable that factors at all levels impinge on the development of individual cases of the condition. Genetic factors determine that some individuals will have a liability to schizophrenia – this predisposition has been called *schizotaxia* by Jacques Meehl (Meehl, 1962). Not everyone who is schizotaxic will become schizophrenic. Adverse conditions in early development, such as birth complications or maternal infection, will exacerbate abnormalities in the developing nervous system of some individuals, increasing their risk, whilst benign conditions may protect other individuals. Later in life, a subset of those still vulnerable will undergo maturational or life stresses which bring on a psychotic episode. Even this is not the end of the story; whilst some patients become chronic sufferers, in and out of hospital and care all their lives, others recover completely from their psychotic symptoms and live more or less normal lives. Those diagnosed and treated early have a higher chance of this outcome. Thus there is another level of risk factors that make a difference to the outcome, that of the social and medical conditions surrounding the patient who has a psychotic episode.

The model of causation for schizophrenia is shown in Figure 3.7. The vertical arrows are pathways leading upwards towards a case of chronic schizophrenia. The arrows can only go on upwards by passing through each of the oval windows which represent the various risk factors for the disease. There are a relatively large number of people with schizotaxia (the bottom level), some of whom also experience difficult neurodevelopmental environments, and life stressors. Some of them have a psychotic episode; even they will only go on to develop the full chronic disorder if their pathway goes through the remaining risk window of inadequate social and medical response. It must be stressed that this model is still somewhat hypothetical, but it is a plausible representation of the causal sequence involved in this most serious psychiatric problem. It shows clearly that just because a disease has a genetic component, it does not mean that the environment is unimportant, or that nothing can be done, since there are many intermediate levels at which an intervention can make all the difference.

Figure 3.7 A possible model of the causes of schizophrenia.

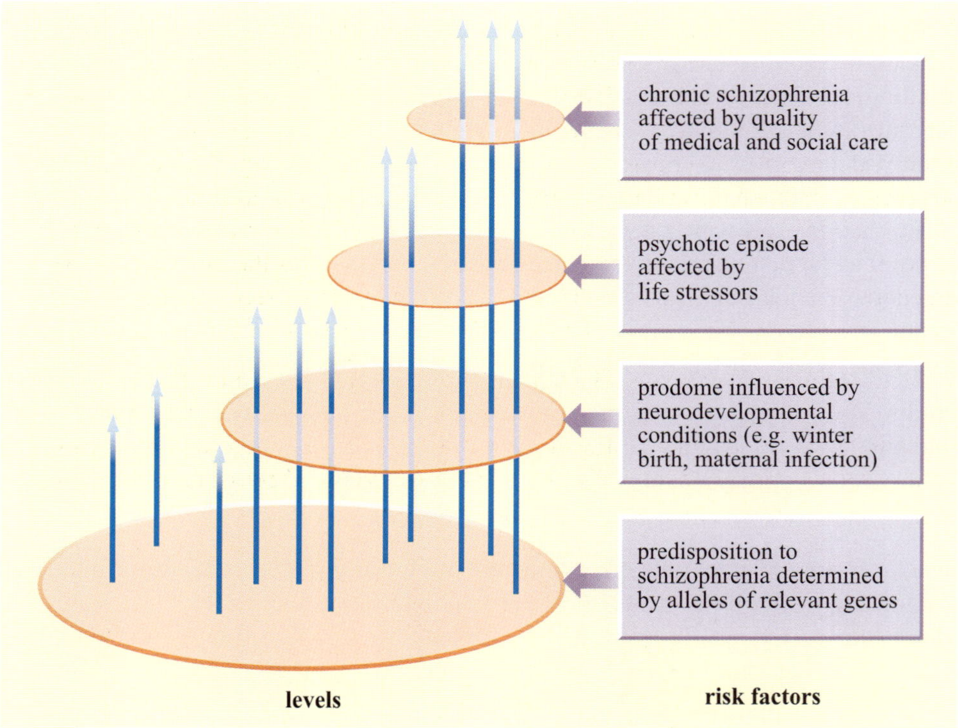

3.5 Recovering from schizophrenia

Until the 1950s, there were no objectively effective treatments for schizophrenia, though this certainly did not stop certain surprising practices like prolonged insulin-induced coma being carried on in psychiatric hospitals. The prognosis of the disease was depressingly poor. The evidence on long-term outcome in the developed countries over the last one hundred years has been put together by Richard Warner (Warner, 1994). Only about 20% of those people who had an episode recovered completely and returned to normal economic, social and family life. Perhaps 40% made a more modest improvement, in the sense that they lived more or less independently. That leaves 40% who became chronically ill and dependent. They could expect to spend long periods compulsorily detained in psychiatric institutions.

Since the 1950s, two great changes have occurred. First, drug treatments have become available for schizophrenia (as discussed in Section 3.3.1), and, second, a trend against institutionalization that began before the Second World War has been continued and has led to a drastic decrease in long-term hospitalization.

As we saw in Section 3.3.1, the first drugs used to treat schizophrenia patients were the phenothiazines, and their close relatives. The therapeutic effect of chlorpromazine and its relatives depends on their ability to suppress the activity of dopamine.

- The phenothiazines and related drugs are called 'antipsychotics'. Why are they not called 'antischizophrenic' drugs?
- The evidence shows that they suppress positive symptoms. There is no evidence that they can undo the neurodevelopmental basis of schizophrenia, and their effect against negative symptoms is less than against positive ones.

Like most psychiatric drugs, the phenothiazines are complex molecules with a chemical structure that acts like a key that fits into the molecular lock of receptors on the surface of neurons. They bind to the receptor, thus either enhancing or blocking its activity. The problem with antipsychotics is that the key fits too many different locks, causing disruption to many parts of the nervous system. For a start, there are several different main dopamine pathways in the brain (Figure 3.8). One of these, the nigrostriatal dopamine pathway, is heavily involved in the control of movement (this is the pathway underactive in Parkinson's disease; Book 4, Section 1.6.4). Activity in this pathway is not thought to be related to psychotic symptoms. However, the phenothiazines affect this pathway as much as the others, and thus can cause a Parkinson's like tremor as a side-effect. (Conversely, levodopa, the dopamine enhancer used to treat Parkinson's disease, can produce hallucinations.)

Worse than this, phenothiazines have many effects beyond those on dopaminergic activity. They also bind to receptors for the other neurotransmitters histamine, adrenalin, and acetylcholine. Each of these bindings causes side-effect problems (Figure 3.9) which can include dizziness and lowered blood pressure, dry mouth, drowsiness, blurred vision and weight gain.

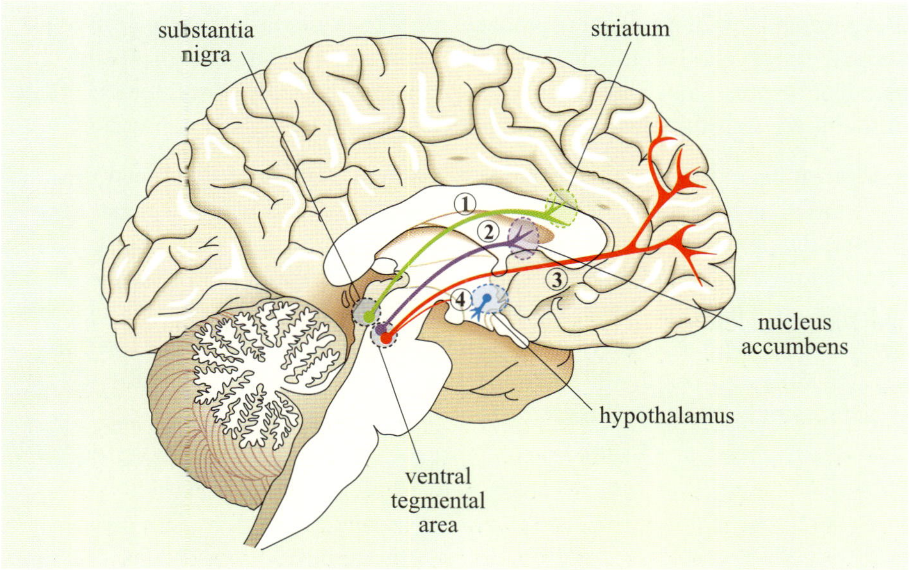

Figure 3.8 The dopamine neural pathways in the human brain. The numbered pathways are as follows: (1) nigrostriatal pathway, (2) mesolimbic pathway, (3) mesocortical pathway, (4) tuberoinfundibular pathway.

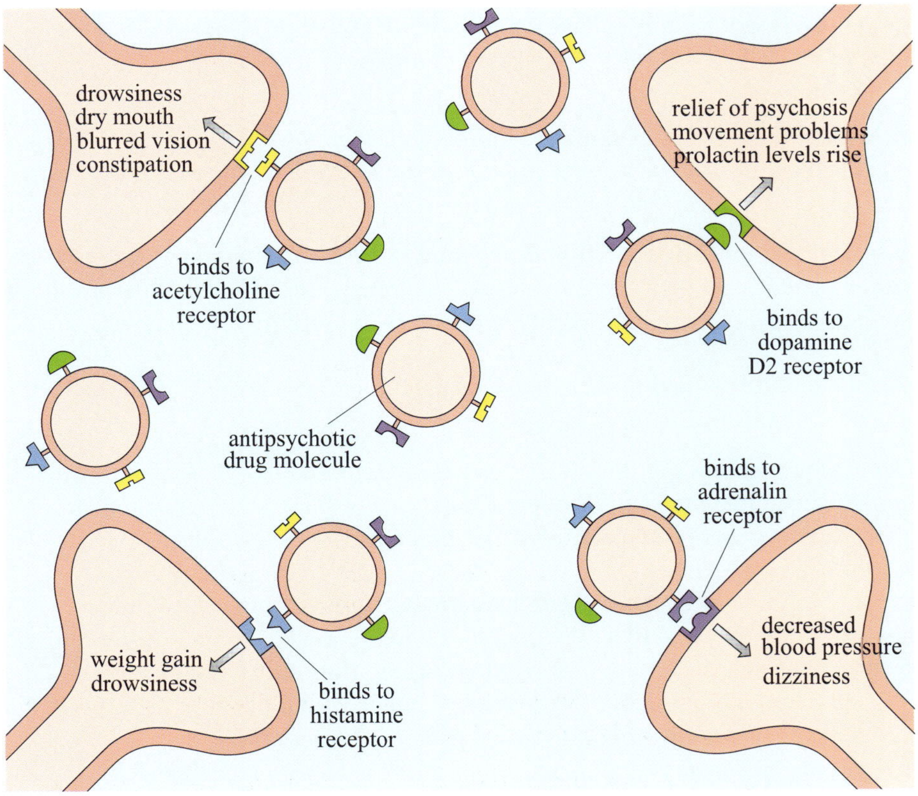

Figure 3.9 Mechanisms of therapeutic action and side-effects of a typical antipsychotic drug such as a phenothiazine.

In view of the problems associated with these 'typical' antipsychotics, the search was on for a compound which would target the desired dopamine pathways specifically and leave the nigrostriatal dopamine pathway alone. Several new generation drugs now exist, and they are collectively referred to as the 'atypical antipsychotics'. They bind more strongly to receptors in the mesolimbic and mesocortical dopamine pathways than in the nigrostriatal one. Thus they cause fewer problems of tremor. They are still quite non-specific in other ways: they interact with all the neurotransmitter systems that the earlier generation did, plus one more – serotonin! However, their side-effect profile is generally seen to be more favourable than those of their predecessors. They are at least as effective as the classical antipsychotics in reducing positive symptoms. There is also some evidence that they can ameliorate negative symptoms, possibly through their effects on serotonin, the transmitter most often associated with mood and depression.

These days we have drug treatments for schizophrenia, but does that mean the prognosis has changed? Sadly, the evidence suggests that it has not changed that much. First, incidences of schizophrenia are roughly stable, and a psychotic breakdown almost always involves hospitalization for a period. Fewer people are now in psychiatric hospitals on a very long-term basis, but we should not take this to mean that they are necessarily having trouble-free lives. It seems that the old ratios – 20% fully recovered, 40% partially recovered, and 40% chronically ill – remain depressingly accurate (Figure 3.10).

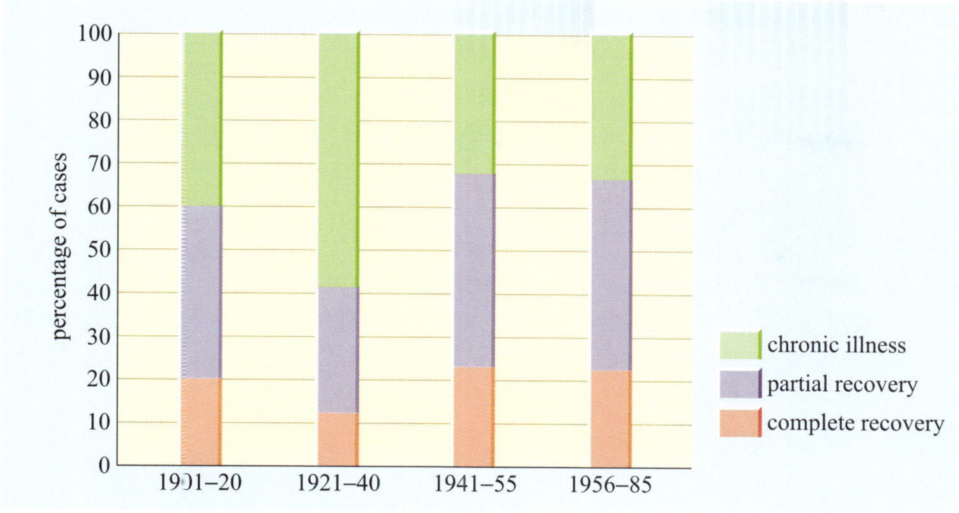

Figure 3.10 Percentage of schizophrenia cases leading to complete recovery, partial recovery and chronic illness, for different periods through the 20th century.

◆ Why might having drugs that suppress positive symptoms not help people very much in terms of work and family life?

◆ It may be that negative symptoms and cognitive problems are just as disabling as hallucinations and delusions in terms of the ability to get on with normal life and relationships.

Can schizophrenia be cured? As we saw in Figure 3.7, the causes of schizophrenia are best understood as a series of influences operating cumulatively at different time points. A drug might one day be developed which will be much more effective at controlling the symptoms that cause people the most trouble. However, as we have seen, some of the prodromes are already present way back in early life. These difficulties are unlikely to be reversed by a drug which an individual only starts taking years later when a psychotic episode happens. It may be that at-risk individuals can be given dietary supplements and neuroprotective agents before any positive symptoms have appeared. There would, however, be serious ethical issues in prescribing drugs with side-effects to people not yet diagnosed with any illness.

◆ Look again at the multifactorial model of the causes of schizophrenia (Figure 3.7). In view of this, are drugs the only innovation which could affect the occurrence and prognosis of schizophrenia?

◆ No – interventions at many levels could all make a difference, from public-health measures that improve maternal health and reduce birth complications, to better diet and less stress amongst young people, to a more enlightened social and medical response to the onset of psychotic symptoms.

Summary of Section 3.5 and conclusions

In recent decades, schizophrenia has been mainly treated with antipsychotics like the phenothiazines. These suppress positive symptoms in most patients by their effect on dopaminergic pathways originating in the midbrain. However, they have low biological specificity and many side-effects. Modern atypical antipsychotics may have fewer side-effects.

Drug treatments have had limited effect on the prognosis of schizophrenia, which remains poor for most people. The possibility remains that medical and public health interventions will ultimately reduce the incidence and improve the prognosis of the condition.

3.6 Normality and disorder revisited

We round off this chapter by revisiting the issue of whether schizophrenia is 'really' an illness or not. In the 1960s and 1970s it was fashionable to argue that it was not. Constructionists argued that schizophrenia was simply a label attached by society to anyone it found too difficult to accept and whose perspective it sought to exclude. Attention was drawn to the fact that in the Soviet Union, the diagnosis of schizophrenia was given to dissidents as an excuse to lock them up and marginalize their voices, and similar examples. This movement cheered the end of large-scale hospitalization, and questioned the need for compulsory treatment at all.

Constructionist arguments were easy to make when there was little evidence on the underlying biology of schizophrenia, but are much more difficult to sustain now. However, we should be very careful of throwing out the baby with the bath water. It is certainly true that there is no abrupt dividing line between the phenomena of 'schizophrenia' and those of 'normality'. Think of the symptoms; emotional flatness, difficulty initiating voluntary acts, unorthodox thinking, distractibility. Who does not recognize themselves in this list, to some extent? Where is the line to be drawn between an eccentric individuality and a diagnosed illness? Even positive symptoms, the diagnostic litmus test, do not provide a neat dividing line. Surveys show that many ordinary people whom no-one would dream of detaining under the Mental Health Act as a psychiatric patient have occasional hallucinations. Sometimes these are to do with stress; they are common, for example, amongst the bereaved. In other cases they become a valued part of life; most cultures have a tradition of hearing voices or seeing signs as part of their religious or spiritual system. Why are these signs of normality whilst schizophrenic hallucinations are signs of 'disease'?

Points such as these are often raised against the biomedical view that schizophrenia is an illness. However, they in fact square rather well with the biological evidence. All these points show is that normal mental life and schizophrenia sit on a continuum with no abrupt gap between them (and a grey area between them instead). But this is precisely what the biological research shows too. Many chemical and anatomical irregularities have been found in schizophrenic brains, but they are statistical differences only, with overlap and continuity between the patients and the control sample. The same holds for the genetic findings; many candidate alleles, but no one allele which is found in all schizophrenia patients but not in any controls.

In other branches of medical research, such a pattern would be taken to indicate that the key biological mechanisms haven't been found yet. For example, cystic fibrosis is caused by the CF allele in the sense that the CF allele is present in a double dose in all and only cystic fibrosis patients. There is no factor for schizophrenia of this sort, which is why many researchers say that the origin of schizophrenia is still a mystery. However, the symptoms of cystic fibrosis are discontinuous from normal physiological functioning in a way that is simply not true for schizophrenia. It is best to see 'schizophrenia' and 'normality' as two overlapping distributions, not two distinct states. Given this view, it may be that we have already found many of the key biological mechanisms, though we don't yet know how they work or which are most important.

In fact, though schizophrenia (the full-blown disorder) is a negative state, schizotaxia (the underlying psychological type) may not be. Many of the most creative and spiritual individuals show certain apparently schizotaxic traits – unusual patterns of thought and behaviour, unorthodox beliefs, a tendency to have visions and hear voices Where this does not become too disorganizing, and where it can be expressed in a socially accepted form such as art or religion, this kind of thing is usually seen as one of humanity's great psychological assets, rather than as an impairment.

So should schizophrenia be termed an illness? Something that differs from healthy functioning only by degree doesn't sit very easily with our usual notion of illness, which is a separate state brought on by a clearly identifiable external factor. But then high blood pressure, depression, arthritis, lumbago and irritable bowel syndrome are all matters of degree, and all the results of multiple causes, and we seem comfortable with the idea that those are illnesses. Moreover, there is the issue of level of control; there is every difference in the world between the occasional hallucination that the subject is able to identify as such, and chronic psychosis.

The constructionists wanted to attack the notion that schizophrenia was an illness, and many of them were genuinely motivated to improve the lot of patients. However, they ignored the most compelling reason for treating something medically, which was human distress. Patients and their families experience enormous personal distress which is not much helped in practical terms by constructionist sociological arguments. Reducing the suffering and suicide associated with schizophrenia requires expensive drugs, research and medical facilities, which governments will not be persuaded to pay for something that isn't a 'real' disease. Arguing that schizophrenia is not an illness but a social construction runs the danger of leaving patients with no support.

3.7 Summary of Chapter 3

Schizophrenia is a spectrum of severe, chronic abnormalities of thought and behaviour. We have reviewed the chemical, cellular and anatomical abnormalities of the brain which are associated with it. We have considered the role of genetic and environmental factors in causing it. We have reviewed some of the main drugs used in treating it, and noted that social and public health factors are likely to affect its incidence and prognosis. Finally, we have argued that both the biology and psychology of schizophrenia lead to the view that it is on a continuum with normal brain functioning. However, it is extreme on that continuum and causes such problems of living that medical intervention is justified.

Learning outcomes for Chapter 3

After studying this chapter, you should be able to:

3.1 Recognize definitions and applications of each of the terms printed in **bold** in the text.

3.2 Understand the symptoms involved in the diagnosis of schizophrenia.

3.3 Describe briefly the different types of biological abnormalities that have been associated with schizophrenia.

3.4 Describe the techniques used to investigate possible brain abnormalities in schizophrenia.

3.5 Describe the different factors that have been implicated in causing schizophrenia, and the evidence for each of them.

3.6 Explain the difference between a linkage study and an association study.

3.7 Describe how genetic and environmental factors might interact in producing a complex psychological state.

3.8 Evaluate the arguments for and against considering schizophrenia as a disease.

Questions for Chapter 3

Question 3.1 *(Learning outcomes 3.1 and 3.2)*

What are the major classes of symptoms of schizophrenia?

Question 3.2 *(Learning outcomes 3.3 and 3.4)*

Review the section on the brain basis of schizophrenia (Section 3.3). Fill in the gaps in Table 3.3, specifying the level of analysis, the abnormality found, or the technique used for finding it.

Table 3.3 For use with Question 3.3.

Level	Abnormality found	Technique for finding or inferring abnormality
Neurochemical	Excess dopamine activity	Inferred from actions of drugs; some studies of HVA levels
Neurochemical	Increased D2 receptor density	
Neurochemical	Increased serotonergic activity	
Neurochemical	Reduced glutamate	
Cellular	Reduced grey matter	
Cellular	Distribution of cell bodies in cortical layers	Examination of post-mortem brain tissue
Neuroanatomical		CT and MRI scans
Neuroanatomical	Relative metabolic activity levels of different brain regions during different tasks	

Question 3.3 *(Learning outcome 3.5)*

For each of the following factors that could play a causal role in schizophrenia, briefly describe the evidence that they do:

(a) genetic factors

(b) parenting

(c) maternal condition at the time of pregnancy and birth

(d) life stress

Question 3.4 *(Learning outcome 3.6)*

Each of these statements describes either linkage studies, association studies or both types of study. Decide which it is that:

(a) Aims to identify genes involved in a specific condition.

(b) Uses individuals belonging to the same family.

(c) Takes biological samples from the participants to discover which genetic variants they have.

(d) Can be affected by irrelevant differences in the genetic composition of the population.

(e) Has to distinguish individuals who have the condition under investigation from those who do not.

(f) Uses unrelated participants drawn from the population.

Question 3.5 *(Learning outcome 3.7)*

On balance, does the weight of evidence suggest that schizophrenia is caused by genetic factors or by factors in the environment?

Question 3.6 *(Learning outcome 3.8)*

There is no single factor that differentiates all schizophrenia patients from all normal individuals. Therefore, schizophrenia cannot be a true disease. Briefly discuss this statement.

CHAPTER 4

CONSCIOUSNESS REVISITED

4.1 Introduction

Doubtless you are feeling a sense of relief at having finally reached the last chapter of the last book of SD226. So, by now, you have earned some time for reflection, not only on the earlier chapters of the present book but on the other books and, if you wish, even on the 'meaning of life' itself! This chapter will not introduce any new material but it will be an opportunity for you to reflect on some of what has gone before, to see new interpretations of the evidence and to form new links between phenomena.

At night, as you drift into sleep, you might well spend time asking such questions as – who am I? What is the essential nature of this conscious human? What makes an individual unique? Do I make free choices or is my behaviour the inevitable outcome of predetermined factors? This kind of question almost inevitably appears when you study biological psychology. We are sorry if you will feel cheated but, in the few pages that remain, we will not be able to provide convincing answers to these questions! However, what we can do is to remind you of where biological psychology is of central importance to their discussion.

As its name implies, this chapter has the intention of revisiting the subject of consciousness. It will do so with a principal focus on the preceding three chapters of this book but will also cast its net wider to cover other books of the course. It will attempt to bring some of the rest of the course together, using the phenomenon of consciousness to do so.

Consciousness was first mentioned in Book 1, Chapter 1, where you were introduced to the idea that biological psychology calls upon at least two sorts of information:

- objective and observable phenomena, such as behaviour and the physiological performance of the brain, and
- subjective reports of the contents of conscious awareness.

Usually only the detached scientist has access to information concerning the performance of the brain, obtained by such means as PET scans of the brain and electrical and chemical recordings from the brain. By contrast, only *you*, as a conscious individual, have access to your conscious mind and can report on its contents. This is termed a 'first-person perspective'.

As you saw in Book 1, Chapter 1, a profound challenge for biological psychology and philosophy alike is to try to account for how to relate these domains. That is, how are the mind, including its conscious aspects, and the physical brain linked? As was discussed, various ideas and analogies have been proposed to explain this association. Needless to say, none of the explanations provides an entirely convincing account. We will shortly return to consider this issue again.

First, the chapter will remind you of some of the more biologically based material on consciousness that was discussed in earlier books of the course. It will then turn to consider Chapters 1–3 of this book.

4.2 Individual cases, brain damage, minds and consciousness

This section is intended to remind you of some famous cases of brain damage that have contributed so much to our understanding of biological psychology. Some of these cases arose through disease or accidents and some through surgery designed to alleviate suffering. Later sections of the chapter will build on the evidence from these cases.

4.2.1 Patient D.B.

As the first case, Book 1, Section 1.1.6 introduced the patient D.B. and the phenomenon known as 'blindsight', which was described further in Book 1, Sections 4.3.4 and 4.4.2.

- Can you recall what the term 'blindsight' means?
- A person with damage to part of the visual cortex can at first appear to be totally blind to events in the part of the visual field corresponding to the damage. However, other evidence points to the retention of some visual capacity.

That is to say, the patient appears blind in terms of a conscious report of not seeing anything. However, by an objective index, the patient can be shown to respond to visual events corresponding to the 'blind' part of the visual field. Patient D.B. showed reactions to stimuli that he claimed not to see. For example, he could direct eye movements to visual stimuli and guess better than chance concerning the form of the visual images.

- What is an important lesson here for studying conscious and unconscious processes?
- A person does not always have insight into all the determinants of his or her behaviour. The conscious report might be saying one thing but an index of behaviour is saying something rather different.

Since D.B. was 'cortically blind' in a region of his visual field and was not aware of 'seeing' visual images associated with this region, this suggests that conscious awareness only arises at the cortical level of processing. You might like to describe the situation in the following slightly convoluted way: in a sense, D.B. knew something about the visual world but did not know that he knew it.

4.2.2 Patient H.M.

As the second case, Book 1, Section 1.1.5 introduced you to the patient H.M., who reappeared in Book 5, Section 1.5.1, and Section 2.5.2 of this book. H.M. had parts of the temporal lobe, including the hippocampus, removed in an attempt to cure intractable epilepsy. In this regard, the operation was successful.

- Can you recall the problems encountered by H.M. following the operation?
- H.M. was unable to update his memory based on the *new* episodes in his life. For example, he would meet the same psychologist over and over again but did not show any sign of recognizing him or her.

The ability to recall episodes of our past experience is surely a fundamental feature of the contents of the conscious mind. The term episodic memory is used to refer to this class of memory (Book 5, Section 1.1.3).

- Was there any aspect of H.M.'s memory that remained intact after the operation?
- H.M. was able to engage in conversation, which required a memory for language and recently expressed ideas. Also H.M. showed intact skill learning over trials: in performing eye–hand coordination in a reverse-mirror drawing task. However, H.M. could not recall having engaged in this task, even though he showed improving skill at it.

As with D.B., patient H.M. is cited as evidence for a fracture line between conscious and unconscious processing. In each case there is evidence for processing carried on at an unconscious level, which does not have access to conscious verbal articulation.

- Can you speculate on the nature of phenomenal consciousness experienced by H.M.?
- Being unable to update his episodic ('personal') memory one might speculate that H.M. lived more in the 'here-and-now' than would an intact control person.

Patients such as D.B. and H.M. provide valuable insight into some of the neural correlates of consciousness (Book 1, Section 4.4), a topic to which we return later.

4.2.3 Split-brain patients

Before considering split-brain patients, let us note first that information presented to the left-hand side of the brain's midline is directed to the right side of the brain, whereas that on the right side is directed to the left side of the brain (see, for example, Book 4, Sections 2.3 and 2.6). However, communication occurs between the hemispheres, such that information received by one hemisphere is normally available to both.

Book 5, Section 2.3.2 introduced the term 'split-brain' patient, to refer to surgery carried out as a treatment for severe epilepsy.

- What does the term 'split-brain' refer to?
- Patients with a surgical cut through the corpus callosum, the large bundle of fibres that link the two hemispheres of the brain (Book 1, Section 1.3.2).

- What is the implication of this intervention regarding processing of information?
- The normal sharing of information between hemispheres is eliminated, or at least severely disrupted.

- Can you recall which side of the brain normally has the prime responsibility for processing information on language?
- The left hemisphere is described as being lateralized for language.

Where a task requires an intact channel of communication between information arriving at the right hemisphere and the language processing regions of the left hemisphere, performance is seriously disrupted in a split-brain patient. For example, a task consists of targeting visual information to the right hemisphere and then asking the patient to describe in words what is seen. Typically, 'nothing' is the response. This is because the left (language) hemisphere does not have access to information from the right hemisphere. However, except on such specific and unusual tasks devised in the laboratory, split-brain patients can appear for the most part to be remarkably normal in their day-to-day behaviour. There are some anomalies though. For example, one hand can start to button up a coat while, at the same time, the other hand proceeds to unbutton it. This points to two separate commands to action arising in the two hemispheres.

The interesting question in the present context concerns whether, in splitting the brain, we have thereby split consciousness. Is it meaningful in any sense to suggest that we have created two conscious selves in one brain? The answer to this is largely speculative. However, in the case of one patient, experimenters were presenting different tasks to the two hemispheres and the patient suddenly remarked – 'Are you guys trying to make two people out of me?'

Having set the scene on brains, minds and consciousness, we will now turn to some of the theoretical issues that cases such as D.B., H.M. and split-brain patients can be used to illustrate.

4.3 Brains, minds, 'easy' problems and the hard problem

4.3.1 Introduction

Book 1, Chapter 1 introduced the topic of how we might relate brains and minds and this was developed further in Book 1, Chapter 4. It was suggested that the mind is 'what the brain does'. Now that you have learned more about brains, their constituent cells and what brains do, you should be in a better position to appreciate such claims. Clearly, as you have seen throughout the course, brains process information. For example, they extract information arriving at the sense organs and they programme motor action in the world. So, are such aspects of the brain 'doing something' included in what we mean by 'mind'? By definition, they have to be included, but such features of information processing do not really capture the essence of the lay use of the term 'mind'. In this sense, it is more commonly used as in, say, 'I simply cannot make up my mind' or 'my mind was so gripped with fear'. In such a context, 'mind' has a more personal, idiosyncratic and emotionally coloured quality.

Perhaps the lay use of 'mind' implicitly refers to the *conscious* mind and, as you have seen, this is also assumed to be one feature of the brain doing something. However, it is not the only feature, since, in various parts of the course, you have seen a number of examples of behaviour being influenced by information processing that remains at an unconscious level. H.M. and D.B. exemplified this, and numerous tests on intact participants told a similar story.

Book 1, Section 1.2.3 introduced the use of analogies in trying to understand brain and mind, so could these clarify the issue? Analogies to the brain have called upon the technology that was current at the time. From our privileged 21st century perspective, the analogy has seemed to improve with the technology. For example, in the first part of the 20th century the brain was compared to a telephone exchange, with incoming and outgoing telephone messages. These days, with the advent of information technology, the computer is the most common analogy. One can hardly even speculate on what tomorrow might bring.

- Can you recall the computer analogy?
- It was suggested that the physical hardware of the computer is analogous in some ways to the brain, whereas the software, the programme running on the computer, is analogous to the mind.

- Is this compatible with the argument that the mind is 'what the brain does'?
- It would seem to be. What the computer does is described in terms of its programming and the kind of operations that it performs.

Such analogies give a tentative first grip on the topic of brains and minds. However, philosophers and neuroscientists are engaged in endless protracted debate on how much the brain is really like a computer. So, never get too carried away with such analogies. They can never be more than first guides to our thinking.

No matter how excellent and rapid a calculator a computer is, how many of you believe that your computer is conscious, i.e. that it has experiences of phenomenal consciousness? Very few people would surely go that far. Yet some scientists do speculate that one day computers will acquire so many features of the human brain/mind that it would be discriminatory not to grant them membership of the club of the conscious. If the brain is indeed a super information processor, and so are computers, what is the barrier to crediting the computer with consciousness? You could even programme the computer to say yes to the question – are you conscious? – so it would respond much like you would (well, so we hope!). This leads us to the so-called hard problem of consciousness.

4.3.2 The hard problem and 'easy' problems

There are certain problems of consciousness, which are relatively easy to solve, or at least we know how to pose the right question to address the problem. For example, we can ask intelligent questions concerning the pathways of information processing that remain intact in the cases of D.B. and H.M. They are not exactly lightweight considerations, you might feel, but nonetheless, we can well imagine the kind of answer that might be obtained, in terms of defined intact pathways of neurons.

Alas, even this ability to envisage the kind of answer that might result is not the case with what is known as the hard problem of consciousness (Book 1, Section 4.2.2).

- Can you recall what the term 'hard problem' means?
- The hard problem is how a state of phenomenal consciousness, involving feelings, can arise from inanimate matter, the material that makes up the brain.

Having studied SD226, you are in a better position to appreciate why the hard problem is indeed so hard. Researchers are now able to record the activity of single neurons or groups of neurons and relate this to behaviour. Brain imaging techniques have enabled us to reveal which brain regions in normal healthy individuals are activated, corresponding to such events as recognizing a face or a word. You saw throughout the course how the workings of the brain are to be explained in terms of neurons and neurotransmitters, etc. The brain, like the rest of the body, is made up of various chemicals, proteins, fats, ions, water, etc. These make up the neurons and glial cells that form the brain. For example, the action potential is explained in terms of the movement of sodium and potassium ions across the neuron membrane (Book 4, Chapter 1). However, in spite of the wealth of such insight into the brain, we still do not know how on Earth the *raw feel* of a toothache or being in love arises from such activity by systems of neurons.

There is nothing in the properties of neurons to suggest that when they are put together to form complex nervous systems, out should pop conscious awareness with all its emotional colouring. How this happens is the hard problem. We cannot answer it here but, as an OU student, please do not feel short-changed because neither can anyone else answer it. As Book 1, Section 4.2.2 noted, there is an *explanatory gap* in our understanding, though you might feel that 'explanatory chasm' or 'gulf' would better convey the truth! What we can at least claim is that, as a result of studying the brain, we are in a better position to formulate the question of how physical processes occurring at the level of neurons are experienced as conscious thoughts. This must seem like a modest claim indeed but we would hope that it is an honest and realistic one.

There is another aspect of the hard problem closely related to that just described. Imagine when you last did something totally spontaneously, i.e. not driven by events happening just prior to the act. You might suddenly decide to sit down or get up for no apparent extrinsic reason. The experience of this is felt to be free. Of course, as Book 4, Section 3.3 described, there are defined motor pathways from the motor cortex via the spinal cord to skeletal muscles involved in such action. However, exactly how a conscious decision arises and is translated into the *instigation* of action remains a mystery.

The term *emergent property* was introduced in Book 1, Section 1.4.3. It might be that this notion could provide the last desperate refuge for the beleaguered psychologist, neuroscientist and philosopher concerned with the hard problem.

◆ What is an emergent property?

◆ It is a property that emerges from a *combination* of components but is not evident in the characteristics of the individual components. The property only becomes evident when they are put together.

◆ Can you recall the example of the liquidity of water as an emergent property?

◆ At room temperature, the gases oxygen and hydrogen do not exhibit liquidity. When oxygen and hydrogen are combined to form water, liquidity emerges from the combination.

The brain doubtless exhibits emergent properties, features that are evident in the performance of complex combinations of neurons but which are evident neither in the behaviour of individual neurons nor in nuclei. For example, the control of movement (Book 4, Chapter 3) requires the delicate interaction of numerous nervous system regions, e.g. cerebellum, motor cortex, basal ganglia and spinal cord. Similarly, Chapter 3 of the present book suggested that abnormalities in just one part of the brain might not be enough to produce schizophrenia. Rather, the combination arising from a slight abnormality in each of a number of regions might be necessary.

So, can the notion of emergent property help with consciousness? It seems likely that consciousness can usefully be described as an emergent property of the combination of billions of cells that makes up the central nervous system. Indeed, what is the alternative? One could speculate that each cell of the body possesses consciousness to some degree, rather as some serious thinkers postulate that every atom of the Universe is conscious, a version of panpsychism (from the Greek for 'all' and 'soul'). As you might have guessed, there are not many biological psychologists amongst the believers of this idea. Also, it moves the problem elsewhere – to finding out how simple matter can be conscious.

Much as we might be inclined to argue that consciousness is an emergent property of the brain, there is a serious problem with this and it amounts to another statement of the hard problem. Even if one acknowledges that the wetness of water is an emergent property, nonetheless a chemist will tell you that, looking at the component gases, there is every reason to expect liquidity to emerge from their combination. Similarly, the neuroscientist accepts as obvious that complex behavioural performance *emerges* from the combination of numerous nervous system components. Neither would he or she be at all surprised that the appearance of a behavioural disorder such as schizophrenia might emerge from abnormality in several places. By contrast, there is nothing in the properties of neurons or their combination that in any way suggests the emergence of conscious awareness. This is indeed hard and, the more that you know about the problem, it seems only to get harder.

Similarly, you might well feel that it is precisely here that the computer analogy breaks down. The analogy might capture the essence of the information processing and give a useful first distinction between hardware and software. However, surely it would be hard to persuade you that, out of those wires and silicon chips, emerges anything even remotely like conscious awareness and feelings. You might well have felt anger towards your computer when the 'stupid thing' loses your TMA but you will hardly ever have felt compassion for it, or have been in receipt of feelings from it, or have you!?

If consciousness emerges from the brain, it is interesting to speculate about the stage of development at which it first emerges. Book 3, Chapter 3 described the development of the brain, noting that we start our lives as a single fertilized cell. So at what age has brain complexity reached a stage that is able to support consciousness? We do not know the answer. It is not very insightful to pose the question to a participant unless a certain age of verbal fluency has been attained!

Book 1, Section 4.3.4 discusses the function of consciousness. What is the functional advantage of having a brain that exhibits this property? Again, this immediately draws the hard problem and the easy problems back into focus. It is easy to identify the kind of tasks that are performed consciously, such as focused attention on pursuing a mate, escaping a predator, reflecting on the future and resisting temptation. It is not hard to see that a capacity to perform such processing gives us a functional advantage. If, however, we ask about the functional advantage of the *experience* of phenomenal consciousness that accompanies such processing, we are back to the hard problem. Why could a brain not achieve all of these processing operations by acting as a zombie? We must again plead modesty here!

The brain does have 'zombie' modes of operating. For example, the eye movements of D.B. towards stimuli were performed with no accompanying awareness, suggesting that this mode of operation is present in all of us. Such zombie modes are rapid, efficient and rather stereotyped. However, to multiply their number indefinitely would appear not to be an economical way of working. It is probably better to have a number of them but to incorporate a flexible conscious mode of operation in the design, which permits thinking and planning.

Book 1, Section 4.2.1 raised the issue of self-consciousness. That is to say, I am not only conscious, i.e. have feelings and phenomenal consciousness, but I am aware that I am conscious. The chapter promised to reconsider this question in Book 6 and to return to the issue of whether this is a uniquely human attribute. Well, we cannot escape it but can we give any insights?

As was noted in Book 5, Section 2.1, humans are not unique in having language. For example, by means of the distinctive vocal calls that they emit, vervet monkeys are able to convey information about different types of predator. However, no species comes near to exhibiting the human capacity for richness of structure and content of language. Therefore, we might speculate (and it can only be speculation) that there is something uniquely human about our capacity for self-awareness. With the help of language we are able to represent the past and the future. We have a self-image as part of our representation of the world, and we can hypothesize about our participation in future worlds or worlds that might never even exist. A highly sophisticated and complex language appears to play a crucial role in mediating our self-consciousness.

Now we are in a position to reconsider some of the issues raised in Chapters 1–3 of this book, relate them to the discussion of consciousness and to see links between topics. A focus now is the neural correlates of consciousness. You might be relieved to know that appeals to modesty and inadequacy can afford to be somewhat less frequent now.

4.4 Motivation

As was described in Chapter 1 of this book, an important feature of motivation is the experience of affect ('hedonic factor'), as a consequence of feeding, sex and drug-taking. In essence, affect is a private (first-person) experience. However, there are behavioural correlates of the experience, and it was even speculated that rats show evidence of affect in their facial reactions. It was noted that endogenous opioids play a role in the hedonic calculation associated with ingesting a food. Blocking opioidergic transmission reduces the hedonic impact of otherwise tasty foods.

- ◈ Have we any reason to suppose that unconscious factors could also play a role in the calculation of the affective value of a food, i.e. how much pleasure is associated with tasting it?
- ◆ Book 1, Section 1.1.6 provided experimental evidence of just such an effect. It described an experiment in which images of happy, angry and neutral faces were flashed onto a screen very briefly, with the time of exposure adjusted such that the participants reported not seeing the faces at all. Participants were then asked to rate the quality of a drink.

- What was the outcome of this experiment?
- The quality of the drink, in terms of amount poured and drunk and the price that the participant reported being prepared to pay for it, was influenced by the subliminal image. The happy face increased the rating of the drink relative to the neutral face whereas the angry face decreased it.

This experiment demonstrated that events that do not gain access to our consciousness can nonetheless have an important influence on our behaviour, suggesting the possibility that opioid levels were affected by the subliminal image.

Related to consciousness, Section 1.4.2 of this book also described craving, as in an addict's intense desire for a drug that is not available. This is a private first-person experience.

- Are there correlates of craving that are open to objective analysis?
- Yes – as was described, in drug addicts, imaging studies reveal increased activity in parts of the brain involved in emotional processing (e.g. the amygdala), when craving is triggered by presenting drug-related stimuli.

4.5 Emotion

4.5.1 Introduction

The central importance of the first-person experience in emotion is evident in the opening words of Chapter 2 of this book:

> 'Emotions! Here is a topic that many people consider should be central to understanding much of human behaviour, for throwing light on our happiness and on our miseries.'

The importance is equally evident when we consider the list of basic emotions given in the chapter: happiness, sadness, anger, fear, surprise and disgust. One might imagine (albeit with difficulty) the existence of these human emotions even in the absence of overt behaviour but it would make little sense to try to imagine them in the absence of first-person feelings.

An important message of Chapter 2 of this book was that each emotion has various characteristic aspects:

1 a particular brain activity

2 activity of the autonomic nervous system,

3 particular types of behaviour that are triggered and

4 states of consciousness.

A complete understanding of human emotion requires a consideration of all of these. Certain non-human animals (e.g. rats) clearly exhibit aspects 1–3. Whether they experience aspect 4 is a matter of philosophical speculation. However, we try to deal with non-human animals and make laws on animal welfare and cruelty on the basis that they have such experience. In their research, biological psychologists often make the explicit or implicit assumption that animals have subjective feelings. This is evidenced by the term 'pleasure centres' introduced in Section 2.4.3 of this book.

- In what sense was this term employed?
- It was used to describe particular regions ('centres') of the brain. A rat in a Skinner box would press a lever and receive a direct electrical stimulus to the centre through an electrode with its tip located there.

- Does this notion of pleasure in rats remind you of anything discussed in Chapter 1 of this book?
- The facial reactions of rats to the application of substances to their tongues are sometimes described as being indicative of an 'affective' or 'hedonic' factor (Section 1.2.4).

4.5.2 Brains and their damage, emotion and consciousness

Insight into the role of conscious and unconscious processes in emotion is of importance in trying to understand brain mechanisms and to assess the effects of their damage. For example, Book 1, Section 4.3.2 and Book 4, Sections 2.2 and 2.5 discussed the phenomenon of prosopagnosia, associated with damage to the inferior posterior temporal lobe of the brain.

- Can you recall what prosopagnosia is?
- It is the condition where a person can recognize a face as being a face but expresses no idea as to whether the face is familiar or not.

- Is this all there is to the phenomenon or do we have reason to believe that at an unconscious level there can be recognition of certain faces as familiar?
- A difference in galvanic skin response is registered between a familiar and unfamiliar face. Skin conductance depends upon the secretion of sweat, which is a measure of emotional arousal.

- What is the possible significance of this result?
- There is an emotional reaction by the autonomic nervous system triggered by the brain acting at an unconscious level.

Concerning the emotion of fear, Book 1, Chapter 4 described two pathways involved in the fear response, with the amygdala playing a crucial role in both. Chapter 2 of this book considered this topic in more detail. One pathway was described as relatively direct and rapid ('better safe than sorry' or 'quick and dirty'), whereas the other was described as relatively slow and indirect. The 'dirty' part of the description refers to the fact that this route is responsible for a relatively simple and crude reaction to gross features of the image, rather than a more refined analysis.

- Can you recall the routes that these pathways took in the brain?
- The quick route was eye → thalamus → amygdala, whereas the slow route was eye → thalamus → cortex → amygdala.

- ◆ What is the assumption regarding the link between these pathways and consciousness?
- ◆ It is assumed that the subcortical pathway is associated with unconscious processing whereas the cortical route is associated with conscious processing.

As was discussed in Book 1, Section 4.3.2, and Section 2.8.2 of this book, an imaging experiment investigated the effect of exposure to subliminal images of happy or fearful faces. This was associated with activation of the amygdala, particularly so in the case of fearful faces. Again, dissociation was found between the subjective report of seeing nothing and an objective measure, activation of the amygdala.

- ◆ Does this remind you of an experiment just discussed under the heading of 'motivation' (Section 4.4)?
- ◆ You should recall the effect on taste reactions of presenting subliminal images of happy and angry faces. In each case, there is an effect mediated at an unconscious level.

Section 2.5.2 of this book considered the role of the hippocampus and amygdala in learning about emotional events. It discussed the case of a comparison between two sets of rare patients; those who have bilateral damage to the amygdala and those who have bilateral damage to the hippocampus. The experiment is directly relevant to the issue of the conscious recall of episodes of experience and the disruption of this capacity. First, conditioning was carried out, in which a tone was paired with a mild shock. The capacity of the tone to trigger a change in skin conductance was then measured. Intact subjects would readily show such conditioning and be able to report on their participation in the conditioning trials. That is to say, they had a consciously accessible memory of the episodes of their experience.

- ◆ What would a reaction to the tone indicative of fear be termed?
- ◆ A conditional response (Book 5, Section 1.2.2). The change in skin conduction is conditional upon the tone being paired with the shock.

In this study, patients with damage to the amygdala showed no evidence of conditioning to the tone as measured by skin conductance. However, they were able to report on the experience of their participation in the conditioning trials. Thus, although they had a consciously accessible memory of the events, those events were not associated with a normal autonomic reaction. Conversely, patients with damage to the hippocampus showed evidence of conditioning, as measured by changes in skin conductance. However, they were not able to recall the experience of being exposed to the conditioning trials.

- ◆ Such a combination of results is described by a particular term that was introduced in Section 1.3.3 of this book. Can you recall the term?
- ◆ A double dissociation. (Lesion x disrupts reaction X but not reaction Y whereas lesion y has the opposite effect.)

- ◆ In what regard do the participants in this study with hippocampal damage remind you of the performance of H.M.?
- ◆ H.M. was unable to recall his participation in the trials of the reverse-mirror task even though his performance improved.

Finally, no concluding chapter in an account of brain and behaviour would be complete without a brief return appearance of Phineas Gage, the unfortunate soul who suffered brain damage in a railroad explosion (Book 1, Section 1.1.4). Gage damaged his frontal lobes and thereafter showed less responsibility and was more impulsive in his behaviour. Chapter 2 of this book briefly reconsidered Gage, noting that he:

> '… became easily distracted and uninhibited in his emotions after damage to his frontal lobes.'

The frontal lobes are involved with planning for the future and resisting impulses that tend to arise in the immediate environment. As such, they are associated with an important aspect of conscious processing. Of course, no one would suggest that Gage lost his consciousness in the years following the accident. Consciousness doubtless arises from the interaction of many brain regions but appears to be able to survive some damage to part of its neural substrate. Unable to talk to him, all we could reliably claim is that Gage suffered disruption to an aspect of information processing associated with consciousness.

4.5.3 When emotions go wrong and therapies to treat them

The study of consciousness is also important in understanding how mood and emotion can go wrong. This can be exemplified by depression. Box 2.6 of this book described the American Psychiatric Association's diagnostic criteria for depression. These are as follows:

1. persistent feelings of sadness or anxiety
2. loss of interest or pleasure in usual activities
3. changes in appetite that result in weight losses or gains not related to dieting
4. insomnia or oversleeping
5. loss of energy or increased fatigue
6. restlessness or irritability
7. feelings of worthlessness or inappropriate guilt
8. difficulty thinking, concentrating or making decisions
9. thoughts of death or suicide or attempts at suicide.

◆ Which of these are in principle observable in terms of behaviour? Which are based exclusively on first-person reports, and which are mixed?

◆ It would seem that insight into factors 1, 6 and 7 can be gained only by first-person reports. Factors 2, 3, 4, 5, 8 and 9 can be derived from both behaviour and first-person reports. In no case, is behaviour alone an index.

Just as considerations of consciousness are vital to understanding emotional disorder, so are they to understanding its treatment. Chapter 2 considered two broad classes of treatment for emotional disorders: chemical interventions in the form of drugs and mindfulness-based cognitive therapy. In cognitive therapy, consciousness, as revealed by first-person reports on thinking, is central. The nature of maladaptive thought processes can be identified and challenged. In the case of drugs, their mode of action is known in targeting particular classes of neurotransmitter in the central nervous system, e.g. the SSRIs (specific serotonin reuptake inhibitors) target serotonin.

- Is the first-person perspective (consciousness) irrelevant when we consider drug therapies?
- Not at all. The rationale is to change thought processes and improve affect, both intrinsically conscious processes. The effectiveness of therapy (or otherwise) can only be assessed in terms of first-person reports by the patient.

As Chapter 2 notes:

> 'Depression is both in the mind and a chemical imbalance. Brain activity on the one hand, and thoughts and feelings on the other, are not two separate items but different aspects of the same highly complex phenomenon.'

To argue which is the most important would be misguided, and this forms one important concluding message for SD226.

4.6 Schizophrenia

4.6.1 Introduction

Chapter 3 of this book described schizophrenia. The consideration of consciousness is of central importance to understanding what the phenomenon is, and how it might be explained and treated.

The positive symptoms of schizophrenia were described in terms of hallucinations and delusions. Our evidence for these derives from the reports by the patients themselves, i.e. as first-person data, in terms of the content of their conscious awareness. Suffering is caused by the abnormality and intrusiveness of such thoughts. For years, people with schizophrenia can suffer in silence in their private world of abnormal consciousness. So, the study of consciousness in psychology clearly matters, not least when it goes so awfully wrong as here.

Section 3.2.2 noted that:

> 'Descriptions of schizophrenia report social withdrawal and problems of coordination, attention, concentration and willed action.'

This might have reminded you of the discussion of the relationship between consciousness and attention (Book1, Section 4.3.3) and motivation (Chapter 1 of this book). The discussion now turns to consider these aspects of schizophrenia.

4.6.2 Attention

As Book 1, Section 4.3.3 observed, the process of attention is closely tied to consciousness. It was noted that 'when people talk about attention, they usually mean conscious focused (or selective) attention'. It was also described how tasks can be performed in the absence of directing attention to them. For example, a skilled driver can carry out routines such as steering, accelerating and gentle braking, even though his or her conscious attention is directed elsewhere, e.g. worrying about the next TMA or talking to a passenger. Hence, there is a system of allocation of attention to the demands of different tasks. Learning consists of building up pathways that link familiar stimuli and their associated responses.

When we try to understand what goes wrong in schizophrenia, insights into attention can be valuable, since evidence points to disturbances to attention. Chapter 3 noted that a feature of schizophrenia is 'disorganized speech (e.g. frequent derailment or incoherence)'. It seems that one feature of this is a disturbance to attention, such that consciousness gets captured by irrelevant stimuli and this breaks up the story-line.

Discussing patients with schizophrenia, Section 3.2.2 noted that:

> 'In one well-studied paradigm, they do not seem to get used to a repeated signal as quickly as control participants do, continuing to show a large cortical response to it even after several repetitions'.

This suggests that conscious processing capacity is being engaged with a signal that would be labelled as 'of no interest' ('redundant') by control participants and thereby handled at an unconscious level.

4.6.3 Motivation

Features of schizophrenia might also have reminded you of Chapter 1 of the present book. The negative symptoms of schizophrenia were described as including avolition (a difficulty in initiating actions by one's own will-power) and affective flattening. Motivational systems were described in Chapter 1 as those which are involved in our active engagement with the world, in selecting a course of action and persisting with it. The chapter described affect as being a consequence of successful engagement with the world, as in tasting a good food. It appears then that something goes seriously wrong with motivation in the case of schizophrenia.

4.6.4 Biological basis of schizophrenia

A consideration of the brain volume of patients with schizophrenia compared to that of controls can also give some pointers to the basis of the disorder and how information processing is disrupted. In patients with schizophrenia, the frontal lobes and the temporal lobes (specifically the hippocampus) are reported to be on average below the size of these regions in controls (Section 3.3.3 of this book). You might recall from Book 1, Chapter 4 that the frontal lobes are implicated in tasks that involve handling novelty, such as in producing behaviour in unfamiliar circumstances, where established routines are not available.

Section 3.3.3 of the present book notes:

> 'In a task where a normal participant has to make a voluntary (willed) executive decision ... there is usually a diversion of blood flow to the frontal lobes, and away from other areas of the cortex. This makes sense, as the non-frontal cortex contains the core areas for immediate sensory interpretation, whilst the frontal lobes are thought to be the seat of complex, planned, voluntary actions'.

Under these conditions, this diversion of blood to the frontal lobes is less evident in schizophrenics.

The mesolimbic dopaminergic system featured at centre stage in the discussion of motivation. It can surely be no coincidence that this system is also an important focus of researchers looking into the biological abnormalities that lie at the basis of schizophrenia. It would be so satisfying if we could present a coherent story, such that the avolition of schizophrenia mapped neatly onto inactivity by the mesolimbic dopaminergic system. Alas, at this stage, this would be a speculative intellectual leap too far. Although successful therapies for schizophrenia are designed to target this dopaminergic system, exactly how they act is still unclear. It might be that they exert a bias in favour of exciting one part of the system (e.g. cortical) relative to another (e.g. subcortical).

As a further argument for a role of disturbed dopaminergic transmission in schizophrenia, there is evidence from drugs such as cocaine and amphetamine, and again reports of conscious awareness are central.

- Can you recall from Chapter 1 of the present book what the action of cocaine is?
- It boosts the activity of dopaminergic systems by, amongst other things, blocking reuptake of dopamine (Section 1.4.4 of this book and Book 4, Box 1.2).

Amphetamine also targets and boosts dopamine transmission. The taking of both types of drugs by non-schizophrenic individuals can trigger hallucinations, delusions and paranoia, which is sometimes difficult to distinguish from schizophrenia.

4.7 Final word

So, as we come to finish this chapter, the conclusions could hardly be clearer: we have some reasonable answers to a few of the easy problems of consciousness but little or nothing to say in answer to the hard problem. We can point to neural operations that are carried out perfectly well at an unconscious level. The obvious ones are operations such as the control of breathing and heart rate. Such inaccessibility to consciousness is probably just as well; try to imagine the utter chaos that would ensue if you had to make conscious decisions on how fast the heart should beat! For another example, you are aware of the outcome of visual perception in terms of conscious images but have absolutely no conscious insight into the neural processing that leads to the images.

When we consider the neural correlates of consciousness, we can point to imaging studies in intact participants and evidence on brain damage as contributing valuable insights. With the use of intact or brain-damaged participants, we can demonstrate the important role of unconscious determinants of our behaviour (e.g. when we are fearful or using subliminal images to affect the pleasure gained from the taste of a drink). As with the evidence of blindsight, the work on fear suggests that the activation of the cortex is a necessary condition for consciousness to appear. Further research will doubtless clarify better this issue. We can present analogies that give some tentative hold on issues of brain and mind. However, alas, we are forced to leave you puzzling over the hard problem of how your conscious awareness arises from that 1.3 kg mass of tissue in your head.

What does all this say about our own feeling of personal agency and freedom? Such feelings are usually closely associated with the contents of our conscious mind and as such reflect another aspect of the hard problem. To what extent we really have free agency and quite what this would mean are hard problems for which there is little insight. Is evidence of determination of behaviour by factors outside our awareness evidence on the limits of our freedom? Some would argue just this but the problems remain daunting.

The evidence certainly points to a number of determinants of our behaviour that are quite outside our conscious awareness. Book 1, Section 4.5.1 noted that conscious awareness often appears on the scene after we have already started to perform an action. This suggests important limitations on our intuitively persuasive notion that we first plan something consciously and then put the plan into action. In one experiment, people were observed to be choosing one from amongst a range of four pairs of identical stockings. After leaving the store, they were asked to justify their choice. Most people gave such reasons as the particular quality of the pair chosen. In fact, most people took the pair to the extreme right of the display but no one actually gave this as their reason. It would appear that we sometimes elaborate and apply a story-line to why we do things, oblivious to the true reasons.

So, is consciousness just a kind of free movie show of little consequence to our actions, which are, in reality, predetermined by forces outside our awareness? That could well be going too far. It is one thing to show that a Wimbledon champion is acting at a speed that cannot be accounted for in terms of conscious control or that shoppers have limited insight into the bases of their choice. It would quite another to suppose that, say, our conscious planning to do future good or bad in the world is quite without any real efficacy.

We hope very much that all this gives you something useful to think about but without keeping you awake at night.

Question 1.1

(a) In a state of sodium depletion, a supply of concentrated sodium chloride is needed to replenish the body.

(b) Gastrointestinal distress disturbs the equilibrium of the body. Avoiding this in the future is in the interests of homeostasis (stability) of the body.

Question 1.2

(a) By its association with the drug, the white arm is transformed into an *incentive*, in that the rat is attracted there. The white arm was previously a neutral stimulus but, by its pairing with drug, it becomes a conditional stimulus, a process of *classical conditioning*.

(b) The rat might exhibit an initial preference for either light or dark, irrespective of drug injection.

Question 1.3

To act as a control against the possibility that it was simply the disturbance that triggered increased food intake.

Question 1.4

In biological psychology, the functional account refers to the emergence of something as a result of the advantage it confers in evolution. Drug taking is abnormal in the sense of not having been 'tested' in this way by evolution. The technology (e.g. syringes, refined drugs) is a feature of modern times and represents a hijacking of brain processes that evolved to serve conventional behaviour. However, in a sense, it might be understood as an abnormal manifestation of a process that serves the animal's interests in terms of conventional motivation.

Question 1.5

Although we are in the early stages as yet, PET scans can be taken of addicts when craving is triggered by presentation of cues associated with drug taking. These might provide a reliable objective correlate of a subjective state.

Question 2.1

The emotions happiness, anger, fear, disgust and sadness are usually considered to be universally recognized. Surprise has also been included by some researchers. These emotions are often named as the 'basic emotions' common to all humans. Researchers have taken pictures and video clips to show to people from a range of cultures, as well as recording from these same peoples, in order to test their theories about universality.

Question 2.2

The physiological response is sometimes called the 'fight or flight' response and it prepares the body for strenuous physical activity by, for instance, increasing the blood flow to the major muscle blocks. It diverts the body's resources so that it is better able to fight or rapidly flee in the face of danger.

Question 2.3

Pathway A is the 'quick and dirty' route, which is sometimes called the 'low road' to emotion and responds rapidly to danger based on fairly crude features of the situation.

Pathway C is the slower, more precise pathway, the cortical route in fear, in which the cortex is involved. It allows more detailed and learnt responses to be mobilized. This is sometimes called the 'high road'.

Question 2.4

The amygdala. This area is composed of a number of different nuclei, which seem to perform different functions. The amygdala is richly interconnected with many other areas of the brain. Damage to the amygdala leads to abnormal responses in some if not all emotion situations. It is an area that is frequently activated during imaging studies of emotion processing.

Question 2.5

A, B, C and D are all rated as leading to more lost life-years than war. Unipolar depression tops the list, with more than three times the number of life-years lost in comparison with war.

Question 2.6

A, B, C and D are listed as symptoms that might determine a diagnosis of depression. Persistent feelings of sadness or anxiety, or loss of interest or pleasure in usual activities, are considered to be primary symptoms, whereas there are a number of other secondary symptoms, including A, C and D. Five or more of these secondary symptoms will be present in someone diagnosed with depression.

Question 2.7

B and D. These items are included in the dysfunctional attitude scale. Scores on this scale have been shown to be altered by the drug *d*-fenfluramine, an antidepressant. Attitudes measured by such scales can also be altered by other psychological treatments, such as cognitive behaviour therapy.

Question 2.8

Cognitive models concentrate on understanding how the range of behaviour displayed in fear and anxiety arises, and also how this might be altered by individual differences in anxiety and past experience. The emphasis is on modelling the behavioural outcomes rather than locating neural pathways. Neurobiological approaches are concerned more with locating the neural pathways, and the hormonal and biochemical elements involved.

Question 3.1

The major classes of symptoms of schizophrenia are as follows:

Positive symptoms

hallucinations: unusual perceptual experiences

delusions: unusual beliefs

thought disorder: unusual or circuitous ways of thinking

Negative symptoms

flattened affect: flat emotions

reduced activity: slow speech and movement

alogia: reduced fluency of thought

avolition: difficulty initiating actions

Question 3.2

The completed Table 3.3.

Level	Abnormality found	Technique for finding or inferring abnormality
Neurochemical	Excess dopamine activity	Inferred from actions of drugs; some studies of HVA levels
Neurochemical	Increased D2 receptor density	Post-mortem analysis of brain tissue; PET scanning with participant injected with radioactive ligand for D2 receptors
Neurochemical	Increased serotonergic activity	Inferred from actions of drugs like LSD; inferred from actions of some antipsychotic drugs
Neurochemical	Reduced glutamate	Inferred from drug actions, plus some post-mortem studies
Cellular	Reduced grey matter	MRI scans
Cellular	Distribution of cell bodies in cortical layers	Examination of post-mortem brain tissue
Neuroanatomical	Enlarged ventricles and other abnormalities of brain size and shape	CT and MRI scans
Neuroanatomical	Relative metabolic activity levels of different brain regions during different tasks	PET scans

Question 3.3

The evidence that factors (a) to (d) play a causal role in schizophrenia is as follows:

(a) Genetic factors

- having a biological relative with schizophrenia increases the risk;
- adopted children's risk is predicted by biological not social parents;
- monozygotic twins are more alike than dizygotic twins.

(b) Parenting

- there is no good evidence for a causal role of parenting in schizophrenia.

(c) Maternal condition at the time of pregnancy and birth

- increased risk of schizophrenia with winter birth;
- increased risk of schizophrenia when the mother is infected with a virus;
- increased risk of schizophrenia when there are birth complications.

(d) Life stress

- there are slightly more stressful life events preceding a psychotic breakdown than in controls who have not had a breakdown.

Question 3.4

The statements given describe either linkage studies, association studies or both types of study.

(a) Both.

(b) Linkage.

(c) Both.

(d) Association.

(e) Both.

(f) Association.

Question 3.5

The weight of evidence suggest that both types of factors play a role, and it may be that combinations of genetic vulnerabilities and environmental factors lead down the pathway to schizophrenia.

Question 3.6

The statement seems to imply that diseases have to have a single, identified biological cause to be real. However, this is not the case. Complaints like back pain and irritable bowel syndrome are the products of multiple factors, and there is a grey area between normal discomfort and actual disease. However, it is worth calling them diseases where the distress they cause justifies medical intervention. The same could be argued for schizophrenia.

Chapter 1

References

Di Chiara, G. (2000) Behavioural pharmacology and neurobiology of nicotine reward and dependence, pp. 603–750, in Clementi, F., Fornasari, D. and Gotti, C. (eds) Handbook of Experimental Pharmacology, *Neuronal Nicotinic Receptors*, **144**, Springer, Berlin.

Robinson, T. E. and Berridge, K. C. (1993) The neural basis of drug craving: an incentive-sensitization theory of addiction, *Brain Research Reviews*, **18**, pp. 247–91.

Rose, J. E. and Behm, F. M. (1995) There is more to smoking than the CNS effects of nicotine, in Clarke, P. B. S., Quik, M., Adlkofer, F. and Thurau, K. (eds) *Effects of Nicotine on Biological Systems* II, Birkhäuser Verlag, Basel.

Further reading

For a good account of motivation that assumes some familiarity with science, see Chapters 10, 12 and 18 of Carlson, N. R. (2004) *Physiology of Behavior*, Pearson, Boston.

For an account that assumes no prior understanding of science, see Chapters 16–19 of Toates, F. (2001) *Biological Psychology: An Integrative Approach*, Pearson Education, Harlow, UK.

Chapter 2

References

Adolphs, R., Tranel, D., Damasio, H. and Damasio, A. (1994) Impaired recognition of emotion in facial expressions following bilateral damage to the human amygdala, *Nature*, **372**, pp. 669–72.

Ax, A. F. (1953) The physiological differentiation between fear and anger in humans, *Psychosomatic Medicine*, **15**, pp. 433–42.

Clark, D. M. (1986) A cognitive approach to panic, *Behaviour Research and Therapy*, **24**, pp. 461–70.

Damasio, A. (1994) *Descartes' Error: Emotion, Reason and the Human Brain*, Putman, New York.

Darwin, C. (1872; 1965) *The Expression of the Emotions in Man and Animals*, Chicago University Press, Chicago.

Darwin, C; Ekman, P. (1872; 1998) *The Expression of the Emotions in Man and Animals*, Oxford University Press, London.

Dutton, D. and Aron, A. (1974) Some evidence for heightened sexual attraction under conditions of high anxiety, *Journal of Personality and Social Psychology*, **30**, pp. 510–17.

Ekman, P. and Friesen, W. V. (1986) A new pan-cultural facial expression of emotion, *Motivation and Emotion*, **10**(2), pp. 159–68.

Ekman, P. and Friesen, W. V. (1988) Who knows what about contempt: A reply to Izard and Haynes, *Motivation and Emotion*, **12**(1), pp. 17–22.

Evans, D. (2001) *Emotion: The Science of Sentiment*, Oxford University Press, Oxford.

Flynn, J. (1967) 'The neural basis of agression in cats', in Glass, D. (ed.) *Neuropsychology and Emotion*, Rockefeller University Press, New York.

Funkenstein, D. H. (1955) The physiology of fear and anger, *Scientific American*, **192**, pp. 74–80.

Gray, J. A. (1987) *The Psychology of Fear and Stress*, 2nd edn, Cambridge University Press, Cambridge.

James, W. (1884) What is an emotion? *Mind*, **9**, pp. 188–205.

Kluver, H. and Bucy, P. C. (1937) 'Psychic blindness' and other symptoms following bilateral temporal lobotomy, *American Journal of Physiology*, **119**, pp. 352–53.

LeDoux, J. E. (1998) *The Emotional Brain*, Simon & Schuster, New York.

Murphy, F. C., Nimmo-Smith, I. and Lawrence, A. D. (2003) Functional neuroanatomy of emotions: a meta-analysis, *Cognitive, Affective, and Behavioral Neuroscience*, **3**(3), pp. 207–33.

Oatley, K. and Jenkins, J. M. (1996) *Understanding Emotions*, Blackwell Publishers, Cambridge, MA.

Oatley, K. and Johnson-Laird, P. N. (1987) Towards a cognitive theory of emotions, *Cognition and Emotion*, **1**, pp. 29–50.

Olds, J. and Milner, P. (1954) Positive reinforcement produced by electrical stimulation of the spetal area and other regions of the rat brain, *Journal of Comparative and Physiological Psychology*, **47**, pp. 419–27.

Schachter, S. and Singer, J. E. (1962) Cognitive, social, and physiological determinants of emotional state, *Psychological Review*, **69**, pp. 379–99.

Simon, H. A. (1967) Motivational and emotional controls of cognition, *Psychological Review*, **74**, pp. 29–39.

Further reading

Calder, A. J., Keane, J., Manes, F., Antoun, N. and Young, A. W. (2000) Impaired recognition and experience of disgust following brain injury, *Nature Neuroscience*, **3**(11), pp.1077–78.

Calder, A. J., Young, A. W., Rowland, D., Perrett, D. I., Hodges, J. R. and Etcoff, N. L. (1996) Facial emotion recognition after bilateral amygdala damage: differentially severe impairment of fear, *Cognitive Neuropsychology*, **13**, pp. 699–745.

Cannon, W. B. (1927) The James–Lange theory of emotions: a critical examination and an alternative theory, *American Journal of Psychology*, **39**, pp. 106–24.

Cornelius, R. R. (1996) *The Science of Emotion: Research and Tradition in the Psychology of Emotion*, Prentice-Hall, Upper Saddle River, NJ.

Hamann, S. B., Ely, T. D., Grafton, S. T. and Kilts, C. D. (1999) Amygdala activity related to enhanced memory for pleasant and aversive stimuli, *Nature Neuroscience*, **2**(3), pp. 289–293.

Hess, W. R. (1954) *Diencephalon: Autonomic and extrapyramidal functions*, Grune and Stratton, New York.

Segal, Z. V., Williams, J. M. G. and Teasdale, J. D. (2002) *Mindfulness-based cognitive therapy for depression: a new approach to preventing relapse*, Guilford Press, New York.

Williams, J. M., Watts, F. N., MacLeod, C. and Mathews, A. (1997) *Cognitive Psychology and Emotional Disorders*, 2nd edn, John Wiley & Sons, Chichester, New York.

Chapter 3

References

Andreason, N. C., Paradiso, S. and O'Leary, D. (1998) 'Cognitive dysmetria' as an integrative theory of schizophrenia: A dysfunction in cortical-subcortical-cerebellar circuitry? *Schizophrenia Bulletin*, **24**, pp. 203–18.

Crow, T. J., Done, D. J. and Sacker, A. (1995) Childhood precursors of psychosis as clues to its evolutionary origins, *European Archives of Psychiatry and Clinical Neuroscience*, **245**, pp. 61–9.

Davidson, M., Reichenberg, A., Rabinotwitz, J., Weiser, M., Kaplan, Z. and Mark, M. (1999) Behavioral and intellectual markers for schizophrenia in apparently healthy male adolescents, *American Journal of Psychiatry*, **156**, pp. 1328–35.

Fuller Torrey, E., Rawlings, R. and Yolken, R. H. (2000) The antecedents of psychoses: a case-control study of selected risk factors, *Schizophrenia Research*, **46**, pp. 17–23.

Gottesman, I. I (1991) *Schizophrenia Genesis. The Origins of Madness*, W.H. Freeman, New York.

Heinrichs, R. W. (2001) *In Search of Madness: Schizophrenia and Neuroscience*, Oxford University Press, Oxford.

Jones, P. B., Rodgers, B., Murray, R. M. and Marmot, M. G. (1994) Child development risk factors for adult schizophrenia in the 1946 British birth cohort, *Lancet*, **344**, pp. 1398–402.

Johnstone, E. C., Crow, T. J., Frith, C. D., Husband, J. and Kreel, L. (1976) Cerebral ventricular size and cognitive impairment in chronic schizophrenia, *Lancet*, **2**, pp. 924–6.

Meehl, J. P. E. (1962) Schizotaxia, schizotypy, schizophrenia, *American Psychologist*, **17**, pp. 827–38.

Szasz, T. (1974) *The Myth of Mental Illness*, Harper and Row, New York.

Thompson, P. M., Vidal, C., Giedd, J. N., Gochman, P., Blumenthal, J., Nicolson, R., Toga, A. W. and Rapoport, J. L. (2001) Mapping adolescent brain change reveals dynamic wave of accelerated gray matter loss in very early-onset schizophrenia, *Proceedings of the National Academy of Sciences of the USA*, **98**, pp. 11650–5.

Walker, E. and Levine, R. J. (1990) Prediction of adult-onset schizophrenia from childhood home movies of the patients, *American Journal of Psychiatry*, **147**, pp. 1052–6.

Warner, R. (1994) *Recovery from Schizophrenia: Psychiatry and Political Economy*, 2nd edn, Routledge, London.

Winoukur, G. and Tsuang, M. T. (1996) *The Natural History of Mania, Depression and Schizophrenia*, American Psychiatric Press, Washington, DC.

Wong, D. F., Wagner, H. N, Tune, L. E., Dannals, R. F., Pearlson, G. D., Links, J. M., Tamminga, C. A., Broussolle, E. P., Ravert, H. T., Wilson, A. A., Toung, J. K. T., Malat, J., Williams, A., O'Tuama, L. A., Snyder, S. H., Kuhar, M. J. and Gjedde, A. (1986) Positron emission tomography reveals elevated D2 dopamine-receptors in drug-naive schizophrenics, *Science*, **234**, pp. 1558–63.

Further reading

Bentall, R. P. (2003) *Madness Explained: Psychosis and Human Nature*, Penguin, London.

ACKNOWLEDGEMENTS

Grateful acknowledgement is made to the following sources for permission to reproduce material within this product.

Cover

Anxiety by Edvard Munch (© Munch Museum/Munch-Ellingsen Group/DACS 2003; Photo: © Munch Museum (Andersen/de Jong))

Figures

Figure 1.1a Stahl, S. M. (1996) Essential Psychopharmacology, Cambridge University Press; *Figure 1.1b* Toates, F. M. (2001) *Biological Psychology: An Integrative Approach*, Pearson Education Limited; *Figures 1.3 and 1.5* From Carlson, N. R. *Physiology of Behaviour*, 2nd edn, Allyn and Bacon, Boston, MA. Copyright © 2004 by Pearson Education. Reprint by permission of the publisher; *Figure 1.4* Le Magnen, J. (1967) 'Habits and food intake', *Handbook of Physiology*, vol. 1, 1967, The American Physiological Society; *Figure 1.6* Berridge, K. C. and Flynn, F. W. *et al.* (1984) 'Sodium depletion enhances salt palatability in rats', *Behavioural Neuroscience*, **98**, no. 4, 1984. American Psychological Association Inc; *Figure 1.7* Toates, F. M. and Rowland, N. E. (eds) *Feeding and Drinking*, Elsevier Science Publishers B.V.; *Figure 1.8* Yeomans, M. R. and Gray, R. W. (1996) 'Effects of naltrexone on food intake and changes in subjective appetite during eating: Evidence for opiois involvement in the appetizer effect', *Physiology and Behaviour*, **62**, no. 1, 1997. Copyright © 1996 Elsevier Science Inc; *Figure 1.9* Carlson, N. R. (1998) *Physiology of Behaviour*, 6th edn, Allyn and Bacon, Boston, MA.; *Figures 1.13 and 1.14* Volkow, N. D., Fowler, J. S. and Wang, G. J. (2002) 'Role of dopamine in drug reinforcement and addiction in humans: results from imaging studies', *Behavioural Pharmacology*, **13**, no. 3, 2002. Copyright © 2002 Lippincott Williams & Wilkins; *Figure 1.15* Liu, I. and Weiss, F. (2002) 'Additive effect of stress and drug cues on reinstatement of Ethanol Seeking: Exacerbation by history of dependence and role of concurrent activation of Corticotropin-releasing factor and opioid mechanisms', *The Journal of Neuroscience*, **22**(18), 15 September, 2002. Copyright © 2002 Society for Neuroscience; *Figure 1.17* Shoaib, M., Swanner, L. S., Yasar, S. and Goldberg, S. R. (1998) 'Chronic caffeine exposure potentiates nicotine self administration in rats', *Psychopharmacology*, **142**, 1999, page 330, figure 1. Copyright © 1999 Springer-Verlag GmbH & Co; *Figure 1.18* Jones, H. E. (2003) 'Oral caffeine maintenance potentiates the reinforcing and stimulant subjective effects of intravenus nicotine in cigarette smokers', *Psychopharmacology*, **165**, issue 3, 2003, page 280, figure 1. Copyright © 2003 Springer-Verlag GmbH & Co; *Figures 1.20 and 1.21* Koepp, M. J. *et al.* (1998) 'Evidence for striatal dopamine releases during a video game', *Nature*, **393**, 21 May 1998, Nature Publishing Group; *Figure 1.24* Eysenck, M. (ed.) *Psychology an Integrated Approach*, Longman;

Figures 2.3a and b Punchstock; *Figure 2.5* Eibl-Eibesfeldt, I. (1989) *Human Ethology*, Aldine de Gruyter, New York. Reproduced by courtesy of Prof. Eibl-Eibesfeldt; *Figure 2.6a* Magnum Photos; *Figure 2.6b* Courtesy of Yvonne Royals; *Figures 2.6c and d* The Associated Press Ltd; *Figure 2.7* Sabbatini, R. M. E. (1997) 'The history of lobotomy', *Brain and Mind Magazine*, June 1997, Center for Biomedical Informatics, State University of Campinas, Brazil; *Figure 2.10* Calder, A. J. *et al.* (2000) 'Impaired recognition and experience of disgust following brain injury'

Nature Neuroscience, **3**, no. 11, November 2000, Nature Publishing Group; *Figure 2.11* Murphy, F. C. (2003) 'Functional neuroanatomy of emotions', *Cognitive, Affective and Behaviour Neuroscience*, **3**(3), pp. 207–33, Psychonomic Society, Inc.; *Figures 2.12, 2.13 and 2.14* LeDoux, J. (1998) *The Emotional Brain*, Weidenfield and Nicolson; *Figure 2.15* Reprinted from *Neuroscience and Biobehavioural Reviews*, vol 23, Fendt, M. and Fanselow, M. S., 'The neuroanatomical and neuroschemical basis of conditioned fear', page 752. Copyright © 1999, with permission from Elsevier; *Figure 2.17* Courtesy of Brian Cox; *Figure 2.22* Hammann, S. B. *et al.* (1999) 'Amygdala activity related to enhanced memory for pleaseant and aversive stimuli', *Nature Neuroscience*, **2**, no. 3, 1999, Nature Publishing Inc; *Figure 2.23* Courtesy of Wayne C. Drevets *Figure 2.24* Magarinos *et al.* (1996) 'Chronic psychosocial stress causes apical dendritic atrophy of hippocampal CAS puramidal neurons', *The Journal of Neuroscience*, **16**(10), 15 May, 1996, Society of Neuroscience; *Figure 2.26* Kierman, G. L. *et al.* (1985) 'Birth-cohort trends in rates of major depressive disorder among relatives of patients with affective disorder', *Archives of General Psychiatry*, **42**, no. 7, July 1985, American Medical Association;

Figure 3.1a Lee, K. H. *et al.* (2001) 'Syndromes of schizophrenia and smooth-pursuit eye movement dysfunction', *Psychiatry Research*, **101**, 2001, Elsevier Science Ireland Ltd; *Figure 3.3* Thompson P. M. *et al.* (2001) 'Mapping adolescent brain change reveals dynamic wave of accelerated gray matter loss in very early-onset schizphrenia', *Proceedings of the National Academy of Sciences in the United States of America*, **98**, no. 20, 25 September, 2001. Copyright 2001 National Academy of Sciences USA; *Figure 3.4* Schultz, S. K. and Andreasen, N. C. (2000) 'Functional imaging and neural circuitry in schizophrenia', Harrison, P. J. and Roberts, G. W. (eds), *The Neuropathology of Schizophrenia*. By permission of Oxford University Press; *Figure 3.5* Silbersweig, D. A. *et al.* (1995) 'A functional neuroanatomy of hullucinations in schizophrenia', *Nature*, **378**, 1995. Copyright © 1995 Nature Publishing Group; *Figure 3.6* Gottesman, I. (1991) *Schizophrenia Genesis*, WH Freeman and Company; and Nettle, D. (2001) *Strong Imagination: Madness, Creativity and Human Nature*, Oxford University Press; *Figure 3.8* Stahl, S. M. (1996) Essential Psychopharmacology, Cambridge University Press;

Boxes

Boxes 2.6 and 3.1 Diagnostic and Statistical Manual of Mental Disorders, 4th edn, 1994. Copyright © The American Psychiatric Association; *Box 2.9* Adapted from Weissman, A. (1980) 'Dysfunctional attitude scale', in Corcoran, K. and Fischer, J. (eds) *Measures for Clinical Practice: A Sourcebook*, (1987; 1994; 2000), Free Press, New York.

Every effort has been made to contact copyright holders. If any have been inadvertently overlooked the publishers will be pleased to make the necessary arrangements at the first opportunity.

INDEX

Glossary terms are in bold. Page numbers in italics refer to items mainly or wholly in a figure or table.